Carnivore Code

The Ultimate Guide to Carnivore
Diet, the Ideal Way to Restore
Our Ancestral Diet That Burns
Fat and Builds Muscle

Fox Wild

© Copyright 2020 - All rights reserved.

The content contained within this book may not be reproduced, duplicated or transmitted without direct written permission from the author or the publisher.

Under no circumstances will any blame or legal responsibility be held against the publisher, or author, for any damages, reparation, or monetary loss due to the information contained within this book, either directly or indirectly.

Legal Notice:

This book is copyright protected. It is only for personal use. You cannot amend, distribute, sell, use, quote or paraphrase any part, or the content within this book, without the consent of the author or publisher.

Disclaimer Notice:

Please note the information contained within this document is for educational and entertainment purposes only. All effort has been executed to present accurate, up to date, reliable, complete information. No warranties of any kind are declared or implied. Readers acknowledge that the author is not engaged in the rendering of legal, financial, medical or professional advice. The content within this book has been derived from various sources. Please consult a licensed professional before attempting any techniques outlined in this book.

By reading this document, the reader agrees that under no circumstances is the author responsible for any losses, direct or indirect, that are incurred as a result of the use of the information contained within this document, including, but not limited to, errors, omissions, or inaccuracies.

Table of Contents

INTRODUCTION 1

CHAPTER 1: TURNING BACK TIME 7

What Is The Carnivore Diet? 7
What Is The Carnivore Diet Based On? 9
What Are The Pros Of The Carnivore Diet? 11
Why Is Protein So Important? 16

CHAPTER 2: MYTHS AND MISCONCEPTIONS 21

Plants Provide Vital Micronutrients 21
Plants Have No Negative Effects on Us 23
Will I Get Scurvy if I Do Not Eat Fruits? 40
Is the Carnivore Diet Safe? 41
When Should the Carnivore Diet Be Avoided? 43
Does Too Much Protein Cause Kidney Damage? 45
Ketogenic versus Carnivore 48

CHAPTER 3: LEVELS OF THE CARNIVORE DIET 53

Level 1 56
Level 2 57
Level 3 58
Post Level 3 58
Number of Meals 59
Adapting to the Change 59
How to Deal With the Symptoms: 62

CHAPTER 4: TRANSFORM YOUR BODY AND YOUR MIND 69

WEIGHT LOSS 69
Protein and Weight Loss 69
Reduced Inflammation 74
Improved Heart Health 77

Higher Testosterone in Men *79*
Increased Mental Clarity, Improved Memory, and Focus 81
Improved Mood and Emotional Stability *83*

CHAPTER 5: RECIPES FOR SUCCESS **87**

How Often Do I Need to Eat on This Diet? *87*
A Complete Guide to Pork and Beef Cuts *94*

MEALS 104
Carnivore Flapjack Patties *104*
Carnivore Breakfast Stack *105*
Bacon and Chuck Stew *107*
Meaty Quiche *108*
Soupy Steak Stew *110*
Pork Loin Carnivore Roast *112*
Carnivore Salmon with Garlic and Cilantro *114*
Shrimp for the Grill *116*
Breakfast Sausage Patties *118*
Feta Chicken Patties *120*
Hickory Turkey Burgers *121*
Chicken Pops *123*
Beef Chuck Roast *126*
Lamb Chops for the Grill *128*
Crispy Beef Liver *129*
Roast Beef Brisket *131*
Broiled Parm Tilapia *133*
Marinated Flank Steak *135*
Carnivore Beef Broth *137*

FREEZER/REHEATING FRIENDLY 138
Carnivore Steak Nuggets *138*
Freezer Breakfast Sandwiches *141*
Beefy Taco Pie *143*
Organ Meat Pie *145*
Herb Roasted Bone Marrow *146*
Chicken Gizzards and Broth *148*
Carnivore Freezer Pizza *150*
Yummy Meatloaf *151*
Cocoa Crusted Pork Tenderloin *153*
Easy Roast Beef *155*

Easy Seafood Stock *157*
Slow Cooker Carnivore Beef Stew *159*
Simple Liver and Onions *161*
Freezer-Friendly Italian Meatballs *163*
Bacon Meatloaf Muffins *165*
Slow Cooker Beef Strips *167*
Fish Nuggets *169*
Chili Cheese Dog Casserole *171*
SNACKS 173
Liver and Bacon Cups *173*
Meaty French Fries *175*
Chicken Chips *177*
Party Paté *178*
Egg Loaf Muffins *180*
Angel Food Cake *182*
Parmesan Tuna Patties *184*
CONDIMENTS 186

CHAPTER 6: A WEEK IN THE LIFE OF A CARNIVORE 191

TIPS FOR MEAL PLANNING 195
FREQUENTLY ASKED QUESTIONS: 198
CARNIVORE SHOPPING LIST 202
Supplements for Carnivores *207*

CHAPTER 7: IMPLEMENTING THE CARNIVORE DIET IN YOUR LIFE 213

CHAPTER 8: THE NUTRITIONAL VALUE OF MEAT 223

CONCLUSION 259

REFERENCES 265

Introduction

"Not eating meat is a decision, eating meat is an instinct."

~ Dennis Leary

"Allison lost 100 pounds and cleared eczema on a carnivore diet, Grant no longer has ulcerative colitis symptoms on a carnivore diet, Doug eliminated migraine headaches on a carnivore diet, Nicole found mental clarity on a carnivore diet, Leandro treated his rheumatoid arthritis on a carnivore diet, and Travis healed his skin and digestion issues on a carnivore diet" (MeatRx, 2020). If these real-life testimonials, stated by real people, with real problems appeal to you, then you are in the right place. Through the carnivore lifestyle, these individuals have changed their lives for the better, and you can too. The above-mentioned testimonials cover just the basic benefits of following the carnivore diet. They are but a small part of the success of this revolutionary way of eating.

Living in constant pain or discomfort due to health problems or struggling to lose weight and build muscle can be hard on anyone, regardless of status, age, or resources. With so many possible solutions that arise through medical, scientific, and dietary organizations, it can become overwhelming to invest your trust into a cure without a definite outcome. Searching for the right fit for your individual goals can be exhausting, costly, and ineffective. However, it is evident that most, if not all, carnivore diet followers have restored their health and overall well-being with this eating plan.

"I have now been on a very strict carnivore diet for 7 months with the occasional keto-friendly salad. Very limited alcohol. My doctors have given me regular blood tests and I had an ultrasound on my organs, all the results were A-okay"- Grant Marceau (MeatRx, 2020).

You might be feeling demotivated or uninspired because of weight gain, or on the road to recovery due to illness or injury, whatever condition your body and mind is in at the moment, rest assured that this book will guide you through this lifestyle change with open eyes, whatever your reason may be for changing your habits. There is no "magic secret" or "quick solution," only anecdotal information and guidelines that will help you to reach your goals. Whether it is to build muscle, lose weight, or live a happier and healthier life. Every chapter is curated to educate and inform you on the necessary steps, requirements, and possible side effects of undergoing such a change in your life.

Carnivore Code is authored by Fox Wild, a fitness trainer in his mid-30's, who lost a considerable amount of weight after switching to the carnivore diet. He is well versed on the subject and has 10 years of committed first-hand experience. Fox Wild has found his passion for helping people to achieve their goals through the carnivore diet. At first, he was a skeptic himself. Yet, after achieving a healthier, leaner body, Fox Wild decided to help others to revolutionize their health and make them feel better than ever with the carnivore diet as their primary source of nutrition. It is his passion to resolve the pain of others by educating them on the diet that substantially changed his life for the better.

The first chapter of the book introduces the concept of the carnivore diet and explains the basic tenets and the foundation upon which it is built. It also touches on the historical basis of the carnivore diet and the importance of protein consumption for the mind and body. Chapter 2 follows with a breakdown of common myths and misconceptions regarding the carnivore diet. It dispels the belief that plant-based diets are vital for human life and highlights the impact that they can have on health in general.

There are three main levels to the carnivore diet, and it is important to follow the structure of these levels to achieve your goals in a sustainable manner. Chapter 3 explains the levels in detail and emphasizes the importance of following these guidelines accordingly. It also explains what is allowed in each stage and provides a simple framework to follow. There are several benefits of following a meat-only diet and so far, there has been no evidence of a meat-only diet being dangerous or unhealthy. Chapter 4 covers the benefits of the meat-only eating plan and what it can do for you in the long run.

The next chapter will provide a variety of recipes that you can use while following the carnivore diet. Since this diet is largely based on intuitive eating and does not require eating a set number of meals, these can be eaten for breakfast, lunch or dinner, based on your own preferences. If you are familiar and comfortable with intermittent fasting, then you may wish to incorporate it into your new carnivore lifestyle. All of the recipes are carnivore-friendly and include the required ingredients, step-by-step directions, and tips for preparation. The recipes are split into 3 sections; meals, snacks, and freezer-friendly. You do not have to necessarily use these recipes, but they will be a great source of inspiration and guidance during your journey.

You will also find a sample two-week meal plan that you can review for guidance when planning your own meals and shopping lists. It is designed for each day to have two meals to be adjusted as needed so that you remain satiated and nourished throughout the day. At the end of Chapter 6, you will find a list of useful cooking utensils and other products that might come in handy for food preparation. The cooking styles in the meal plan are merely recommendations and you can use whichever cooking methods, preparations, and styles that you prefer, as long as you stick to the overall guidelines of the carnivore diet. The final chapter provides advice on how to transition to a carnivore diet without too much difficulty. It targets common complaints and difficulties that people have reported, so that you will be fully equipped to handle the food preparations independently.

It is important to remember that changing your life for the better is not an easy thing to do. There will be bad days and it will take some time before you fully adjust to the lifestyle. You will realize soon after starting that, before you start following the food plan, your body is extremely dependent on carbohydrates and/or sugar for energy. When you begin reducing/eliminating carbohydrates and sugar, there may be some unpleasant side effects. However, you will find a lot of useful coping strategies and insight to combat them incorporated into the information in this book.

It is no secret that the carnivore diet receives a lot of scrutiny from plant-based enthusiasts, and they have every right to form their own opinions. However, the truth is in the testimonials of thousands of individuals who have truly lived and experienced the diet for themselves. In this book, you will find more than enough evidence and detailed information regarding what to expect from the diet and how it all weaves into the well-being of the human body and mind. There is much research to be done, but the general take from the carnivore experience is that it promotes a healthy, primal, and organic way of life.

Chapter 1:

Turning Back Time

What Is The Carnivore Diet?

The term, "carnivore diet" is quite self-explanatory. The diet focuses mainly on feeding and nourishing the body with animal products and animal by-products. These products consist of protein-rich foods like meat plus a small intake of dairy products and eggs. Fish is also included in the diet, despite the fact that it is not exactly considered a type of meat. The carnivore diet is an exceptional way of eating because it eliminates all of the unhealthy and processed fats and replaces them with natural, healthy fats and proteins that are usually found in meat products. When you do decide to take on this sort of dietary change, it is important to choose your meat efficiently and carefully. Meat that contains a fair amount of fat can maintain and even boost your energy levels. Whenever you do purchase meat or fish, it is always wise to do so from a trusted butcher who can provide you with high quality products. As well, processed meats are not considered to be as healthful and keeping it organic as possible is always better. Feed your body, and it will feed your mind.

The diet does not include plant-based products like fruits, nuts, vegetables, legumes, grains, or seeds. This might sound strange, considering the popularity of these products among other diets and healthy-eating guides, but the main source of nutrients is not necessarily plant-based foods, contrary to popular belief. The same goes for dairy products that are low in lactose. It is better to go for the purest forms when it comes to dairy products, and it is considerably healthier to eliminate dairy products from your diet entirely. When you look at the ingredients list on products, it is recommended to choose those with the fewest number of ingredients. This may not always be the case, but it is helpful while you are still incorporating dairy products into your diet. Keep in mind that you are trying to mimic the eating habits of our ancient ancestors and they did not have access to processed foods.

To put it simply, the carnivore diet is an all-meat, low-carb diet. The main source of nutrients will be the meat that you consume. Choosing organic, well cut, and fatty meats will help you to maintain energy levels, curb cravings, and stay fuller longer. Maintaining proper hydration is also helpful. An amount equal to about 8-10 glasses daily is recommended. A lot of us confuse hunger with thirst, so drinking sufficient amounts of water can make you feel fuller longer. We are here to feed and nourish our bodies without the toxicity that comes with most foods we choose to consume in these modern times.

What Is The Carnivore Diet Based On?

Our ancestors who roamed the tough terrain and vastness of the savannas of Africa approximately two million years ago instinctively began to add meat to their diets to make up for a detrimental downfall in the quality of plant-based foods. It was this new meat diet, filled with densely-packed nutrients that aided in human evolution, specifically the development and growth of the brain, according to Katharine Milton, an authority on the primate diet. Without eating meat, it is not likely that proto humans could have maintained sustainable energy and nutrition from the plants in their environment to evolve into the dynamic, companionable, and intelligent creatures that they became. In certain parts of the world where the population has little or no access to meat, they have motioned the dangers of malnutrition (McBroom, 1999).

UC Berkeley professor, Tim White, stated that early human genus were hunting, butchering, and consuming animal meat for ages; to be specific, for as long as two and a half million years. Milton claims that animal products like meat provided these early humans not only with all of the required amino acids, but also with vital nutrients as well as integral vitamins and minerals. While protected against nutritional deficiency by consuming meat more often than plant-based foods, our human ancestors could also increase their intake of plant foods with toxic compounds such as cyanogenic glycosides, foods that other primates and animals would have avoided, claims Milton. These compounds are able to yield a fatal amount of cyanide in the body, but this intoxication is defused by methionine and cystine, a sulphur that contains amino acids present in meat (McBroom, 1999). What this information shows us is that our early ancestors and their consumption and utilization of meat played a large, if not massive, role in human evolution. This also proves that meat was, and still is, essential and plant-based foods are merely useful as condiments or extras. Surely, some plants are beneficial to our health, but meat is conclusively a primary source of nutrients.

To summarize, ancient humans lived exclusive on meat from the animals that they hunted and butchered themselves. Carbohydrates derived from plants were mostly supplemental and plant-based foods did not feature heavily in their diets. By utilizing meat as a main food source, early humans were digesting a higher amount of nutrients than they would have if they consumed plant-based foods only. Over several million years we have evolved in many ways; however, we have not evolved to the point where our digestive systems can handle highly processed foods, especially grains and certain vegetables. Meat eating was essential in the development of the human brain and our body uses the energy and nutrients that we gain from it.

What Are The Pros Of The Carnivore Diet?

Weight Loss

Similar to the ketogenic diet, not taking in carbs keeps your blood sugar on the lower side at all times. You will not have insulin spikes, so your body will not feel the need to store calories as body fat. Furthermore, the limited options of foods that you can consume makes it extremely difficult to consume a calorie surplus without resolute effort. This means that you will have to try extremely hard to overdo the amount of calories you consume before you burn them right off again. It is, however, important to understand what the right amount of calories is according to your height, weight, body type, and age.

It is important to consider the fact that, even though you will be losing weight and dealing with a more restricted food list, you will be unlikely to feel or become extremely hungry. This is because fat and protein make us feel satiated for longer due to the tremendous amount of nutrients in the food. If you have a tendency to snack on sugary treats and junk food, then you will still crave it every now and then; however, this is not due to hunger or depravity, but because sugar is highly addictive and can be quite difficult to drop from a diet.

The carnivore diet is also an efficient way to beat the mindless snacking and eating habits that you may have accumulated over the years. Mindless eating and snacking causes the consumption of hundreds, if not thousands, of calories without us even really noticing. Most people develop the habit of eating only when they really have to, once they are on the carnivore diet. This is a very natural way of nourishing our bodies, similar to the habits of our ancestors.

Cardiovascular Health

According to Hyson (2020) a 2013 study in the journal Metabolism compared people who ate a high-fat, low-carb diet to those following a low-fat, high-carb diet. Calories were restricted in both groups of subjects but the high-fat eaters had lower indicators of systemic inflammation after 12 weeks. As a result, the researchers established that high-fat eating, like the carnivore diet, can be more favourable to cardiovascular health. Just by cutting plant foods from your diet you are able to lower inflammation independently.

Less Inflammation

According to Brian St. Pierre of Precision Nutrition, food sensitivity to certain plants then you most likely also suffered from low-level inflammation and when you cut it out of your diet, you are more likely to feel a lot better. He also stated that there is some evidence that eating more gelatinous proteins or foods can improve cartilage health. This is found in products like bone broth, gelatine, and collagen. All of these are components included in most meat products (Hyson, 2020). A lower level of inflammation can result in less tender or fewer sore joints. This means that more meat in your diet can amount to less pain and inflammation in your body.

Digestive Care

Even though we have been led to believe that eating more fiber will result in a more efficient digestive system, it is important to remember that this may not be the case for everyone. Products rich in fiber, like bran and others, have been marketed as the solution to digestive issues for years. Other foods, especially plant products, are often pushed by dieticians and other experts to induce better digestion; however, this is once again, not the case for everyone. The reason why fiber-filled eating could be troublesome for digestion is not clear or concrete, but many reprimand certain components found in plant foods as the main providers of digestive problems. According to the book The Plant Paradox, by Steven R. Gundry, M.D., the natural resistance methods that plants contain to discourage predators may cause bloating, gas, and other digestive issues. These may actually be unsafe for consumption by humans. Lectins, gluten, and phytic acid commonly found in fruits, greens, beans, grains, nuts, and other plant-based products can contribute to inflammation in the stomach and auto-immune disorders such as Irritable Bowel Syndrome, Leaky Gut, and more (Hyson, 2020).

Mental Clarity

Proteins, abundant in meat products, optimizes and elevates brain function and is critical for transferring nutrients to the brain cells in order to nourish and maintain healthy and fundamental heart and brain balance. Protein also aids in the regulation of the brain which is crucial for the modern human's thinking capacity. With the carnivore diet, you can heighten your brain's ability to heal your body, fight off illness, disease and invading bacteria. It also functions as an aid to mental clarity, fights fatigue, and increases your memory (Roberts Stoler, 2015). Protein works wonders for the body and mind, and that is why so many who have had the carnivore diet experience have reached a point of satisfaction in their journey. It does not only work for your body and your desired appearance, but also assists you mentally.

The carnivore diet has been reported as a means to clearer thinking and improved focus, the effects of which are felt almost immediately. However, there is a transition period involved where your body learns how to fuel and nourish itself without carbohydrates. At first, you will most likely experience some lethargy and moodiness. Some also experience mild insomnia and foul breath which is an early indication that your body is going into ketosis, which also means the weight loss and detoxification period is starting. This is no cause for alarm and it is manageable with proper hydration and rest. After the first few days or weeks, you will feel sharp as a tack. You will also start to experience higher energy levels and be able to get more out of your day than you would have before switching to the carnivore diet.

Convenience

The carnivore diet is arguably the least complicated and daunting diet in existence. It is an extremely basic and convenient eating regimen that provides many benefits. It relieves the constant battle with calorie counting, macronutrient tracking, food weighing, and the tedious tasks often involved in other diets. You can start by eating one piece of meat (about 1 lb) in the morning and another during lunch. Some also substitute their meat with eggs or other animal products to keep things interesting. Intermittent fasting is also beneficial, but not obligatory. The diet is simple to follow and your shopping list will be less overwhelming and extremely simple to create. The concern around the high cost of the diet is inaccurate if you consider the fact that meat keeps you satiated for longer, can be stored in the freezer, and will make up for the cost of throwing away fruits and vegetables a few days after purchasing them due to spoilage. In conclusion, it is estimated that it costs more to replace fresh carbohydrates or plant foods every other day than investing in something more sustainable like meat products.

Why Is Protein So Important?

Keeps You Satisfied

The three macronutrients; fats, carbs, and protein, affect your body in different ways. Studies show that, out of the three, proteins are (and always will be) the most filling. They make you feel fuller without having to eat too much. This is due to the fact that protein lowers your level of the hunger hormone known as ghrelin. Protein also enhances the levels or amounts of peptide YY, another hormone that makes you feel satiated longer.

These impacts on your appetite can be quite life changing and astonishing. According to a study by Gunnars (2019), increased protein consumption from 15% to 30% of calories, enabled overweight women to eat 441 fewer calories every day without restricting their calories. People who need to lose weight, especially belly fat, should definitely look into replacing some of their carbs and fats with protein. As we already know, this can be done quite easily when following the carnivore diet, due to the high amount of protein consumption experienced daily.

A food or snack craving is not the exact same thing as normal hunger. It is not about your body needing energy or nutrients, but more about your brain needing a reward or gratification. Cravings are significantly hard to control or get rid of. The best way to get rid of them may be to not let them start festering in the first place.

One of the most effective methods to prevent cravings is to increase your daily protein intake. A study done in overweight men displayed that an increase in protein consumption to 25% of calories reduced cravings by 60% and the desire to snack at night in half. The same was shown in a study in overweight young girls; a high-protein breakfast reduced cravings and late-night snacking. This may be due to an increase in dopamine, a main brain hormone involved in cravings and substances addiction (Gunnar, 2019).

Builds and Repairs Bones and Muscles

Protein acts as a crucial building block of bones, muscles, cartilage and skin. Additionally, your hair and nails are made up mostly of protein. This means eating a suitable amount of protein will enable you to preserve your muscle mass and it also promotes muscle growth during cardio and strength training. Frequent studies show that eating an abundance of protein and mainly protein can increase muscle mass and strength considerably. If you are physically active, lifting weights, or trying to gain muscle, you have to keep a close eye on your protein intake as this could be of great help to you. Adding more protein to your diet will also prevent the disheartening effect of losing muscle when you lose weight. Losing weight is good if you maintain a suitable muscle mass and lose fat, but it is never good to lose muscle. Protein is also needed for repair and recovery. Our bodies use protein to build and repair tissue, which heals the body and promotes the expansion or building of muscles.

One persistent myth preserves the idea that protein (the type that comes from animals) is not good for your bones. This is based on the notion that protein promotes acidity in the body, which ends up sucking the calcium from your bones in order to reduce the effects of the acid. In fact, the longest-standing studies show that protein (like animal protein), is extremely crucial for bone health. According to Gunnar (2019), people who eat higher amounts of protein are able to maintain bone mass more sustainably as they become older and have a reduced risk of osteoporosis and fractures. Women who are at high risk of osteoporosis after menopause should keep this in mind. Eating plenty of protein, staying active, and perhaps following the carnivore diet are all trusted methods for preventing inferior bone integrity. Protein, unlike fat, is not stored in the body and should therefore be consumed quite frequently for it to do its job.

Lowers Blood Pressure

High blood pressure is the main cause of heart attacks, strokes, and chronic kidney disease. Adults with poor eating habits tend to suffer from high blood pressure which can have an extreme impact on your overall health. High protein diets have been known to lower blood pressure and help prevent these diseases from becoming a reality in many people's lives. Research shows that in a review of 40 organized trials, an increase in protein intake or consumption actually helped to lower systolic blood pressure by 1.76mm Hg (on average) and diastolic blood pressure by 1.15 mm Hg. Another study also found that a diet that contained a hefty amount of protein reduced LDL cholesterol or "bad" cholesterol and triglycerides, which is a form of fat that is not necessarily welcome in our bodies (Gunnar, 2019). It is helpful to know that protein also helps our bodies to oxygenate; it supplies our entire body with the nutrients we need to function on a daily basis. Protein also helps with the breakdown of foods and in the generation of production of cells in our bodies.

Complete and Incomplete Proteins

According to Harvard Health Publishing (Fetters, 2020) all animal-based foods, like meat, dairy, and eggs, contain complete protein. Most plant-based protein sources, such as whole grains, legumes, seeds and nuts, spinach, broccoli, and mushrooms, are classed as incomplete. It is widely believed that incomplete protein sources have zero of the nine critical amino acids; however, that is not entirely the case, according to Abbie Smith-Ryan, PhD, CSCS, Director of the University of North Carolina in Chapel Hill's Applied Physiology Laboratory. Many incomplete protein sources have a small amount of every single essential amino acid, just not in levels high enough for that protein to accomplish anything critical. Leucine, which is a main driver of muscle building, tends to be relatively low in most incomplete sources of protein, like vegetables and grains, claims Constance Brown-Riggs, RD, CDCES, who's based in Massapequa Park, New York.

If you regularly eat meat and a lot of other animal products, you will get enough of all of the essential amino acids you need. Most populations in the Western world already consume a lot of meat, which is arguably a very good thing for the overall health and nutrition of these populations. The most recent recommended daily allowance for protein is 0.8 gram (g) per kilogram of body mass. Although, various recent studies, including an article published in July 2015 in Applied Physiology, Nutrition, and Metabolism, suggest more—up to twice that amount—is critical for optimal muscle health, especially in older adults and those trying to lose weight, build muscle, and improve certain health conditions or illnesses (Fetters, 2020).

That being said, the carnivore diet is solely based on complete proteins because our bodies can extract more nutrients from complete proteins than incomplete proteins. This does not mean that plant products are inherently useless as they do hold some sort of nutrient value; however, it is somewhat insignificant when compared to complete proteins otherwise known as animal products. This is why you will often come across claims that vegan and vegetarian lifestyles require a range of supplements to be taken to make up for the lack of complete proteins that are consumed.

Chapter 2:

Myths and Misconceptions

Plants Provide Vital Micronutrients

Many cultures have lived comfortably off of only animal foods for years and some modern people have been following a form of the carnivore diet for decades with no signs of bad health or health issues. The human body requires 10 essential vitamins, essential fats, bioavailable proteins, minerals, and water. Humans do not require any carbohydrates (sugar, starch, and fiber) and do not need micronutrients that come in plants, contrary to popular belief (Roberts Stoler, 2015). If enough proteins and fats are added to your diet, then a lowered amount of dietary carbohydrates is actually a healthy choice seeing that carbohydrate intake has no compatibility with or significance to your quality of life.

The amount of carbohydrates that adds to the human body's optimal health is unknown. This means that there is no true amount of plant-based products that you can consume that will amount to a positive change in your health or your body. According to Heinbecker and Du Bois (1928), there were many traditional populations who consumed a high-fat, high-protein diet that contained only a small amount of carbohydrates for extended periods, like the Masai who are known for their warrior-like stature and behaviour. In many cases, they would live like that for the rest of their lives as did the Alaska and Greenland natives, Inuits, and Indigenous Pampas people. There was no significant effect on health, age, or ability. According to Heinbecker and Du Bois (1928), Caucasians who followed the same diet principles, also handled it quite well seeing that it responded well to their bodies naturally.

It has been proven that other species like rats and chickens can grow and age quite well on a carbohydrate-free eating regimen, but this is only possible if an adequate amount of protein and glycerol from triacylglycerols is present in the diet as substrates for gluconeogenesis (Roberts Stoler, 2015).

It has also been presented that rats actually thrive on a 70% protein, carbohydrate-free diet, which is an important fact to remember seeing that other species also thrive on fewer or no carbohydrates as long as there is enough healthy fat and protein involved. Azar and Bloom (1963) also claimed that the nitrogen balance in adult humans consuming a carbohydrate-free diet needed approximately 100-150 grams of protein daily to survive. Whenever more protein is consumed, other benefits can be received, like the fact that most protein-based products are packed with nutrients that act as building blocks for our minds and bodies. This just underlines the fact that the belief of the myth that plants provide essential nutrients remains challenged.

Plants Have No Negative Effects on Us

According to a trusted Subreddit created for people who follow the carnivore diet (Plants - Zerocarb, 2010), there are multiple anti-nutrients and toxins found in plants that can trigger certain health problems like inflammation, autoimmune dysfunction, and many more. It has even been said that there are endocrine and immune disruptors contained in certain plants that can be quite dangerous when consumed.

Below, you will find tables that give a detailed description of the negative effects of some plant foods (Plants - Zerocarb, 2010):

Anti-Nutrient	Foods	Neutralization	Negative Effects
Phytic acid	Bran of grains and pseudograins, all kinds of seeds, nuts, legumes, potatoes.	Birds and ruminant animals: phytase enzyme. Partly by soaking, cooking, fermenting, sprouting.	Binding with minerals of food in the gut: deficiency of iron, zinc, calcium, and other minerals. Reduces the digestibility of starches, proteins, and

			fats.
Lectins	Grains, pseudo-grains, seeds, nuts, legumes, nightshade vegetables, diary, eggs.	Cooking with seaweeds and mucilaginous vegetables (okra). Partially by soaking, boiling in water, fermenting, sprouting. Wheat, soy, peanuts, and dried beans are	Leaky gut, neurodegenerative disease, inflammatory diseases, infectious and autoimmune diseases, blood clotting.

		the most resistant to neutralization.	
Saponins	Legumes, pseudo-grains, potatoes, red wine.	Different results in studies for soaking, cooking, and fermentation. Cholesterol and bile.	Leaky gut, disturbs digestive enzymes.

| Oligosaccharides | Legumes | Other animals: alpha-galactosidase. Sprouting, fermentation. Bacteria in the colon. | Gas production. |

| Oxalates | Grains bran, nuts, soy, spinach, rhubarb, Swiss chard, chocolate, black tea, some fruits, and vegetables. Metabolite of fungus and dysbiotic flora. Metabolism of the amino acids glycine and serine, vitamin C and sugar. | Partially by cooking. | Binding with calcium: Calcium and magnesium deficiency, kidney stones, disturb digestive enzymes. Hyperoxaluria may play a significant role in autism, COPD/asthma, thyroid disease, fibromyalgia, interstitial cystitis, vulvodynia, depression, arthritis. Researchers believed that "Oxalate hyperabsorption may be the main reason for stone formation in more than half |

			of the idiopathic calcium oxalate stone formers."
Cyanide	Beans, manioc, and many fruit pits (such as apricot kernels and apple seeds).	Cooking and phase II liver detox.	Cerebral damage and lethargy.

Canavanine	Alfalfa sprouts.	Cooking and phase II liver detox and kidneys.	Abnormal blood cell counts, spleen enlargement, Lupus (if a large amount of juice sprouts is taken).
Goitrogens	Soy, peanuts, and cruciferous vegetables.	Cooking, fermenting.	Hypothyroidism.
Tannins	Legumes, some fruits and vegetables, tea, chocolate, wine, coffee, vinegar	Tannin-binding salivary proteins. Partially by soaking and cooking. About 90% by germinati	Zinc and iron deficiency, decrease in both growth rate and body weight gain, perturbation of mineral absorption, inhibition of digestive enzymes,

		on.	accelerate blood clotting, produce liver necrosis.
Trypsin inhibitor	Grains and legumes.	Partially by cooking, sprouting.	Growth inhibition and pancreatitis.
Alpha-amylase inhibitor	Grains, legumes, nuts skin, stevia leaves.	Partially by cooking, sprouting.	Dysbiosis (candidiasis). Deleterious histological changes to the pancreas.
Allicin and mustard oil	Onions, shallots, leeks, chives, scallions, and garlic.	Cooking and phase II liver detox.	Bad breath, and bad body odor, indigestion, acid reflux, diarrhea, stomach pain, gas, anemia, reduced blood

			clotting of open wounds., allergic reactions, accidental abortions in humans. Disturbs a baby's ability to breastfeed.
Salicylates	Berries and dried fruits, some vegetables, herbs, and spices.	Sulfotransferase enzyme.	Same as medicines (aspirin): bleeding of the stomach and gastrointestinal tract, dyspepsia, skin reactions, liver toxicity, prolonged bleeding time, impaired kidney function, dizziness, mental confusion, allergic

			reactions.
Calcitriol, solanine, nicotine	Green potatoes, eggplant, peppers, tomatoes, goji berries.	Liver and kidneys.	Calcinosis, muscle pain and tightness, morning stiffness, poor healing, arthritis, insomnia gallbladder problems.
Gluten	All wheat, rye, and barley plants.		Digestive problems, leaky gut syndrome or autoimmune disease, allergic reactions, and cognitive problems.

| Chaconine | Corn and plants of the Solanaceae family. | Partially by cooking. | Digestive issues. |

Fiber

Macronutrient	Foods	Negative Effects
Fiber	All natural and unprocessed plants and mushrooms	Diverticular disease, constipation, hemorrhoids, bloating, anal bleeding, abdominal pain, leaky gut syndrome, inflammatory bowel diseases, a host of other autoimmune diseases, bowel cancer, depletes vitamins and minerals from the body

Endocrine Disruptors

Endocrine Disruptors	Foods	Negative Effects
Phytoestr	Soybeans	Accelerated aging process,

ogens	and soy products, tempeh, linseed (flax), sesame seeds, wheat berries, fenugreek (contains diosgenin, but also used to make Testofen®, a compound taken by men to increase testosterone). oats, barley, beans, lentils, yams, rice, alfalfa,	androgen hormone imbalances, autoimmune disorders such as lupus, breast tenderness, cervical dysplasia, difficultly losing weight, early onset of menstruation, endocrine imbalances, low male sex hormones, fibrocystic breasts, fibromyalgia, gynecomastia (or "man boobs"), infertility in men and women, irregular menstrual periods, low sperm count, low sex drive/libido, endometriosis

	mung beans, apples, carrots, pomegranates, wheat germ, rice bran, lupin, kudzu, coffee, licorice root, mint, ginseng, hops, bourbon whiskey, beer, fennel and anise, red clover (sometimes a constituent of green manure).	

| Exorphins | Gluten-containing cereals are a main food staple present in the daily human diet, including wheat, barley, and rye. | Gluten intake is associated with the development of celiac disease (CD) and related disorders such as diabetes mellitus type I, depression, and schizophrenia. However, until now, there is no consensus about the possible deleterious effects of gluten intake because of often failing symptoms even in persons with proven CD. Asymptomatic CD (ACD) is present in most affected patients and is characterized by the absence of classical gluten-intolerance signs, such as diarrhea, bloating, and abdominal pain. Nevertheless, these individuals very often develop diseases that can be related with gluten intake. Gluten can be degraded into several morphine-like substances, named gluten exorphins. These compounds have proven opioid effects and could mask the deleterious effects |

of gluten protein on gastrointestinal lining and function. Here we describe a putative mechanism, explaining how gluten could mask its own toxicity by exorphins that are produced through gluten protein digestion. The precise pathway leading to the development of ACD still needs to be discovered. However, the putative mechanism presented in this review could explain this intruding phenomenon. The incomplete breakdown of the gluten protein, resulting in the presence of gliadin peptides with opioid effects, makes it plausible to suggest that the opioid effects of gluten exorphins could be responsible for the absence of classical gastrointestinal symptoms of individuals suffering from gluten-intake-associated diseases. Moreover, the partial digestion of gluten, leading to DPP IV inhibition, could also account for the

| | | presence of extra-intestinal symptoms and disorders in ACD and the occurrence of intestinal and extraintestinal symptoms and disorders in CD and NCGS patients. If so, then individuals suffering from any of these conditions should be recognized in time and engage in a gluten-free lifestyle to prevent gluten-induced symptoms and disorders. |

Immune Disruptors

Immune Disruptors	Foods	Negative Effects
Gliadin	Barley, buckwheat, durum wheat, bulgur, wheat bran,	Incidentally, antibodies to gliadin are capable of binding to nervous system tissue and may contribute to immune-mediated neurological impairment, such as cerebellar ataxia and gluten encephalopathy. Gliadin, particularly the omega fraction, is

	wheat germ, triticale, quinoa, millet, spelt and teff.	also responsible for allergic responses, including Bakers' asthma and the odd wheat-dependent, exercise-induced anaphylaxis (WDEIA).)
Thaumatin-Like Proteins	Fruits, wheat, vegetables, nuts, etc.	Allergies, stimulate immune system, or disrupt physical barriers

DNA/RNA Binding Molecules

DNA/RNA Binding Molecules	Foods	Negative Effects
Rice miRNA	Rice	Alter transcription of LDL-receptor

These detailed analysis tables of the anti-nutrient composition of different plant foods shows us why most of them can be inflammatory and/or harmful to the human body when they are consumed in large amounts, and to those who are particularly sensitive to even low amounts (Plants - Zerocarb, 2010). This just proves how we overestimate the nutritional value of plant foods without considering the toxicity or negative impacts they may have on our bodies.

Will I Get Scurvy if I Do Not Eat Fruits?

A lot of people believe that they will likely suffer from Scurvy which is a side-effect of low vitamin C intake. Although this might be the case in other restrictive diets, it will most likely never occur when you are following a healthy eating plan based on the principles of the carnivore diet.

There seems to be an alternative biochemical pathway for avoiding scurvy that happens when we are eating a fat-burning ketogenic/carnivorous diet, as opposed to a sugar-burning glucogenic diet. While the mechanism of action is not completely obvious, it is believed to be a highly reclaimed fact. Dr. Stephen Phinney (La Fleur, 2015) has hypothesized that the blood ketone beta-hydroxybutyrate may itself be the antiscorbutic component.

According to Gary Taubes (La Fleur, 2015), the vitamin C molecule has almost the same composition as glucose and other sugars in the body. It is carried from the bloodstream into the cells by the same insulin-based moving system used by glucose. Glucose and vitamin C compete in this cellular-uptake process, like two strangers trying to get the attention of a taxicab at the same time. Because glucose is more favorable in the 'contest' the uptake of vitamin C by cells is "globally inhibited" when blood sugar levels are heightened. As a result, glucose regulates how much vitamin C is consumed by the cells. If blood-sugar levels are increased the cellular uptake of vitamin C will fall accordingly. Glucose also weakens the re-absorption of vitamin C by the kidney meaning that the higher your blood sugar is the more vitamin C will be lost in your urine. Concluding that an all meat diet or a low-carbohydrate diet, will bypass the need to consume plant foods that are high in vitamin C.

Is the Carnivore Diet Safe?

Yes, it is completely safe and sustainable. There is no proof that a meat-based diet causes any nutrient deficiencies or harm to the mind or body, but instead, the exact opposite. According to Mike Sisson (2020), an expert on the Primal food and lifestyle movement, carnivore diets blend the benefits of ketogenic and elimination diets together, both of which are already common and well-known for dealing with and treating problematic health problems. An A-Z carnivorous diet is extremely nutritious and provides bioavailable vitamins and minerals, sufficient protein, and other nutrients that the body and mind need. The carnivore diet will also likely put you in ketosis (which may seem unpleasant, but not dangerous) and you will get the anti-inflammatory advantages of ketones, mitochondrial biogenesis, increased fat-burning stages, reduced appetite and cravings, and many more benefits.

Like many other diets, the carnivore diet can be challenging. It is hard to get rid of all the toxins in your body because the detox/ketosis stage is quite hard for some. Surely, there are some arguments that stand against eating this way and it might not be sustainable or possible for everyone, although the benefits it yields does make for a compelling ideology. It should be noted that this lifestyle change requires commitment and sacrifice, but these changes do not put you in danger and you should always listen to your body when you are committed to changing your life.

By removing potentially problematic plant foods, carnivore diets contain little or no FODMAPs, oxalates, lectins, phytates, glycoalkaloids, and salicylates, which are all toxins present in the consumption of plant-based foods (Sisson, 2020). The carnivore diet also offers itself to intermittent fasting and caloric restriction, both of which have remarkable health benefits. Though some may argue that the carnivore diet is too restrictive, high-fat, or other profound lies, it is simply not true based on the evidence we have gathered so far. If ancient humans not only survived, but thrived, on these low-carb diets, then why can't we? This is a question that simply can not be answered factually by those who are opposed to this type of lifestyle.

FODMAP - short chain CHO that are poorly absorbed in the small intestine

When Should the Carnivore Diet Be Avoided?

According to (Streit, 2019), the carnivore diet may be unsuitable for some. In a perfect world, we would all be in peak condition and be able to eat whatever we want. However, due to certain conditions, illnesses, or biological reasons, not everyone can reap the benefits of the carnivore diet. It is unfortunate, but there are other alternatives that may be more beneficial to those who cannot take on the carnivore diet. It is always a good idea to check in with your general practitioner or another medical expert whom you trust before you approach any form of dieting or lifestyle. What works for others, might not work for you.

Those who suffer from chronic kidney disease are not suited for the carnivore diet due to their need to limit their overall protein intake. As you may already know, the carnivore diet is highly focused on an abundance of protein which is beneficial for some, but not for everyone.

Chronic kidney disease, also known as chronic kidney failure, defines the regular loss of kidney function. The kidneys have to filter out wastes and excess fluids from the blood, which are then expelled in the urine. Unfortunately, when chronic kidney disease reaches an advanced stage, dangerous levels of fluid, electrolytes, and wastes can build up in the body. This will deteriorate the overall function of the kidneys and overwhelm the whole system and it is often not detected until the kidney function is significantly endangered. Treatment for chronic kidney disease is based on reducing the advancement of the kidney damage, usually by regulating the underlying cause. Chronic kidney disease can result in end-stage kidney failure, which is deadly without artificial filtering (dialysis) or a kidney transplant (Mayo Clinic, 2019).

People who are more sensitive to the cholesterol in foods, or cholesterol hyper-responders, should be cautious about consuming high-cholesterol foods. The carnivore diet consists mainly of animal foods, which means that it may be high in saturated fat and cholesterol. Saturated fat can raise your LDL (bad cholesterol) significantly when you are already someone who struggles with or is sensitive to cholesterol (Streit, 2019). It may be best then to try a different alternative that offers the same benefits as the carnivore diet.

The same goes for people who are experiencing a condition or illness that has a specific set of required nutrient needs. Children are not well suited for the carnivore diet because their bodies and minds are still in the developmental stage. Pregnant or lactating women should also steer clear as it is not a recommended diet for the first few months after pregnancy and not allowed during pregnancy. Once you are not pregnant or lactating anymore, you can consider switching to a carnivore diet with the proper guidance. Lastly, people who tend to have anxiety about food or have issues with restrictive eating should not try this diet (Streit, 2019). Whether comorbidities were gained through an eating disorder or otherwise, this type of eating should either be avoided or be carefully monitored by a medical expert.

Does Too Much Protein Cause Kidney Damage?

Almost any and all foods contain a certain amount of protein, the only exception being isolated fats and sugars (foods that contain little or no animal byproducts are mostly isolated fats and sugars). Except for those two, the foods with the highest protein masses are largely animal foods. Although animal foods are most likely the best and most bioavailable sources of protein, some plant foods can be high in protein as well. However, we did previously conclude that this protein will not make up for the toxins also found in plant foods. Some may assume that there is a maximum quantity of protein that our body can handle all at once. But this is not exactly true. Evidently, there is no comprehensive limit that concludes the precise amount of protein that everyone can digest or consume. For example, some claim that 30g of protein per meal is the general requirement; however, it is yet to be proven and therefore, not realistic.

According to Joseph (2019), the rate of muscle protein synthesis is at its peak for the first 20-25 grams of protein in a serving or meal, yet we can consume more. The evidence for how much more is not entirely obvious at this stage, but we do know that the recommended intake is higher than previously stated. One particular study that is evidential for this claim was a randomized study examining the effect of a 40-gram beef protein meal versus a 70-gram beef protein meal on protein synthesis in human subjects. In this specific study, the 70-gram serving of beef protein preceded a significantly larger anabolic response. Moreover, all subjects had higher plasma amino acid concentrations than those who consumed the 40-gram serving (Joseph, 2019).

There are relations between high intake and health problems, so for some who ate "too much" protein, there were some problems present. However, there were also associations with improved health in other subjects found in other studies (Joseph, 2019). It is important to remember that these studies were observational, and that the protein intake might be connected to health problems, but that does not mean that they are the cause of the health problems. These studies do not conclude that a high-protein intake leads to more health problems, or any health problems whatsoever.

With that in mind, it is difficult to determine whether it was the protein or the consumption of junk foods that caused the health problems. Someone who consumes more junk food like hamburgers is likely eating a large amount of protein. That does not necessarily mean that the protein in that meal is causing any harm. According to Joseph (2019), a systematic review of 64 prior studies that passed various quality checks concluded that links between a high-protein diet and cancer, cardiovascular, and other health issues were all inconclusive.

As our body digests protein, the process generates a variety of nitrogenous waste components such as urea, uric acid, creatinine, and hippuric acid. These waste components need cleaning out of the body for elimination, and this is the purpose of our kidneys. This process requires a lot of intense effort, which is not abnormal for the kidneys; they collect and process approximately 1.2 liters of blood per minute. This amount accounts for around 25% of all cardiac output, which shows the significance of the kidneys. If waste components build up in the body, they tend to become toxic, and so the kidneys play a crucial role in processing and eliminating these components. This is why so many believe that a high-protein intake can cause kidney strain due to the intense workload that the organ has to endure.

According to the evidence though, high-protein intake does not cause damage to the kidneys. Although it was hypothesized that long-term high-protein intake would create some side effects, clinical trials on human subjects do not condone this hypothesis. Recently, there have been studies that examined this topic, and they all concluded that there is no link between protein intake and alarming signs of kidney health. However, some people who struggle with pre-existing kidney disease or problems should keep an eye on their protein intake (Joseph, 2019). There is currently no evidence that concludes that a certain level of protein consumption is linked to damaging the overall health of our kidneys. This means that there is no such thing as "too much" protein connected to the functioning of this organ and that it should not be considered as a cause for kidney damage.

Ketogenic versus Carnivore

The carnivore diet is often referred to as the most complex version of the ketogenic diet because it permits the consumption of protein and fat, but cuts out plant-based carbohydrates which are allowed on the ketogenic diet. This basic principle sets the two apart quite prominently and to some, it is easier to go full ketogenic before attempting the carnivore diet. This makes sense, seeing that you would then gradually start cutting out plant-based carbohydrates and the effects of a "detox" or the "keto-flu" might not initially be as severe.

Zero Carb

The ketogenic diet generally allows you to have a maximum of 20 grams of carbs daily, where the carnivore diet allows absolutely zero carbohydrates toward the end of the three levels. This is because the end goal is to maintain a diet that is strictly based on the concept of eating only meat, and ultimately, only red meat.

High Protein

The ketogenic diet insists that you keep the protein to a modest level, and fat usually makes up 60-75% of the diet. The carnivore diet, however, consists of primarily protein and the right balance of fat. This is mainly backed by scientific evidence that shows how our bodies are not able to produce protein on their own, and therefore, protein should be one of the main nutrients that we consume daily in order for our bodies to thrive and function properly.

No Carbohydrates

Some vegetables like broccoli, asparagus, Brussels sprouts, and avocados are allowed on the keto diet and are strictly not allowed on the carnivore diet. Even if there is a small adjustment period during your first level of the carnivore diet, it is important to only consume a small number of plant-based foods once a day. If this is still too difficult for you to maintain, then consider going full keto before you move on to the carnivore diet.

Restricted and Advanced

As you already know, the carnivore diet is a restricted and complex version of the ketogenic diet. That being said, it almost completely dismisses the idea of sweet snacks or desserts. The ketogenic diet is considerably more lenient regarding these sweet treats because you can have keto-friendly fat bombs, candies, milkshakes, etc. The carnivore diet does have room for similar desserts, and the amount of sugar should just be taken into consideration. Feel free to flip to the recipe section (Chapter 5) for a delicious angel food cake that is a perfect example of a carnivore-friendly sweet treat.

Different Focus

Maintaining ketosis on a carnivore diet is possible, but it is not the main focus, or a priority for that matter. Your main focus should be on what your body tells you. If you are hungry, eat. If you are full, stop. Your main goal, toward the end, will be to eat your way to a meat- and water-only diet. People on the carnivore diet should not be worried about counting calories or accentuating macros. You are advised to eat until you are completely satiated.

There are two main factors that the ketogenic diet and the carnivore diet have in common. High-fat content and low-carbohydrate consumption are the two key factors that should be considered when approaching both lifestyle choices. That is also why you can easily borrow recipes, ideas, and other tips from the ketogenic diet while you are on level one or two of the carnivore diet. The ketogenic diet consists of high-fat, and the carnivore diet also involves maintaining a healthy balance between protein and fat, and that is exactly why you will be able to maintain ketosis even when you are on the carnivore diet. During the first levels of the carnivore diet (which are explained in the next chapter), you will notice that a small amount of carbohydrates are still permitted, so the ketogenic principles are still somewhat relevant during this stage. Just be careful to not overdo it, as it will make the adjustment period considerably worse.

Chapter 3:

Levels of the Carnivore Diet

Before you adopt this new way of eating, it is important to strategize and set up goals for yourself. Old habits die hard, and as you probably already know, it can become quite exhausting to talk yourself out of 'cheating' when you are on a diet. Luckily, the carnivore diet is more of a lifestyle change than a diet, and it requires commitment in order to be successful. Following the carnivore diet will become easier as you go, but right at the start, you will feel challenged and it will not necessarily be easy.

Dieting and the way you think about it affects different parts of your life because your body acts in response to the information that your eating habits and food intake give it. Every time you eat, you not only boost your protein and healthy fat levels, but you also submit information to your whole body that determines what your next step will be. Your hormones, stomach, and metabolism are calculating what to do with the nutrients that they have received. Your body is programmed to handle the carnivore diet efficiently because it is deeply set in the foundation of your evolution as a human.

This way of eating, or new lifestyle, has some principles that you can follow in order to kick-start your journey to ensure that you experience success. Whatever your reason may be for adopting this new plan, you can always count on these principles to soothe any doubts that you may have. Some of these might seem pretty obvious, but you will be surprised how often we disregard the concepts that should be embedded in our eating habits:

Stop eating when you feel full or satiated: You will find that, like many others, you tend to overeat. Once you start listening to your body, you will realize how often you mindlessly overeat. You might just be surprised.

Simplicity is key: Do not overdress your food. The products used in the carnivore diet are already rich in nutrients and flavor on their own. There is no need to complicate matters. There are a lot of ways to prepare your food deliciously without the add-ons that you are used to.

Stick to animal products: At first this might sound a little scary; however, you should keep in mind that meat, dairy, and eggs are part of our evolutionary diets. Try to consume more red meats instead of white meats and fatty meats over extra lean meats. This also helps to curb cravings and pesky hunger pangs. It does not have to be a costly lifestyle; look out for specials and different ways to save money at your local butcher. You will also feel the need to eat less often, so there is no need to overspend. It is also recommended to eat from one to three meals a day.

Incorporate seafood into your diet: Try eating seafood or fatty fish every other day. If you switch it up regularly, then you are less likely to give into cravings. Get creative with it and try to make the cooking process less of a chore and more of an activity.

Consume other animal products too: If you do not have issues with eggs, as some do, you can incorporate them into your meal plan. Eggs are a great source of protein and they also make you feel full for quite some time. Heavy cream, cheese, butter and ghee are also great products that can ease you into the carnivore diet. Try to avoid milk as much as you can, since it contains sugar. Remember that low-fat or reduced-fat products are not always the best option.

Use salt and pepper: Salt and pepper are a great way to flavor your food without using dodgy seasoning that might contain sugar or other bad ingredients. If you do use spices, try to keep them as organic as possible and remember to check the ingredients label for anything that might hinder your progress.

Do not eat and drink at the same time: Your body will digest your food a lot better when you keep eating and drinking activities separate. Drinking a lot of water throughout the day will prevent you from becoming 'hungry' all the time. We often confuse hunger with thirst and it is always best to hydrate your body.

Stick to low-sugar drinks: Let's be real. No one enjoys drinking water 24/7. Whenever you do consume something else, make sure it is extremely low in unnecessary carbs and sugars. Zero sodas and carbonated water is great every now and then. When it comes to alcohol, you should always keep in mind that the sugar contained in it might be a problem. For the best results, stick to liquor, lite beer, or dry wines. They are lower in carbs and sugar, but think twice before overdoing it. Black coffee with some heavy cream is also a great beverage and energy booster.

There are three levels of the carnivore diet that you should follow as closely as possible with the above principles in mind:

Level 1

During Level 1, all meats, animal by-products, eggs, cream, butter, and cheese is allowed. Level 1 is there to ease you into the diet so that you do not become overwhelmed straight off the bat. You will feel the effects of toxins leaving your body once you are a few days in. Be sure to stay hydrated and focused on your body's signals during this stage. You will find out rather quickly what and how much your body is able to process during the first level. There is no time limit and you can stay on this level as long as you are comfortable with it. If you move to the next level too quickly, the process might become too overwhelming or difficult.

Level 2

Start by removing non-meat products and highly-processed meats from your diet. This means that you should now remove meats like pastrami, salami, and ham as well as any dairy products. Salt and pepper are still allowed, but avoid using too much. The goal is to take another step toward your end goal and become a true carnivore like our ancestors were. Eggs are still fine at this stage, but remember that the end goal is to consume meat and water only toward the end. This is a great time to experiment with seasonings, flavors, cooking styles and eating patterns. You will notice the difference between the two levels almost immediately, but this level can be considered as a pivotal time to determine what works for you and what does not. Do not overwhelm yourself by thinking of what comes next and give yourself time to settle into this level before you even consider moving on to Level 3. It will not always be easy, but if you remain committed to changing your life, the determination will overpower the fear or resistance. Trust the process and you will be more than just fine.

Level 3

All the levels are quite tough at first, but Level 3 is the toughest for most. During this level, you will only be eating beef. All cuts and organ meats are recommended and if it is possible, stick to grass-fed beef. Now is the time to put your experimenting to good use. By this time, you will already notice a big change in yourself. Just stick to the levels and the principles and you will thrive. It also helps to familiarize yourself with your local butcher and keep an eye out for good deals. This does not have to be an expensive lifestyle.

Post Level 3

This is the time where you allow your body to settle into a carnivore diet, as your digestive system and energy levels will need some time to normalize. Do not be alarmed when this takes a little time. However, do not forget to check in with your energy and focus levels. You can also start to re-introduce some things from Level 2. Do this slowly so that your body can adjust without freaking out. Try to remain in each level for about 30 days. Remember, it is a marathon and not a sprint. The carnivore diet is not a quick fix and it will take time and patience.

Number of Meals

This can vary day to day and level to level, based on how you find your body reacts to your new eating habits. The carnivore diet does not require calorie tracking or strict measurements, and has no requirements for how much you should eat per day. Just make sure to stop eating once you are full. If you had success with intermittent fasting previously, or if you are familiar enough with it, you can incorporate it while following the carnivore diet. However, if you are not as accustomed to it, then it is best to stick to three meals per day.

Adapting to the Change

According to Dr. Kevin Stock (2018), your body will respond in various ways once you start your carnivore journey. These changes can be signifiers that your body is starting to adapt to the change and although it might be really difficult, your body will get used to it and the detoxification symptoms will be something from the past. These symptoms can occur when your body is experiencing a carbohydrate restriction phase and it is starting to get rid of addictive agents, chemicals, and other toxins that are still present in your body. The most documented symptoms include, but are not limited to:

- brain fog
- headache
- chills
- digestive issues
- dizziness
- irritability
- bad breath
- dry mouth
- sugar cravings
- nausea
- diarrhea
- frequent urination

To understand exactly what is happening with your body, it is important to look at the various changes that your body is going through during this stage (Stock, 2018).

Fluid Rebalancing

Since you are not eating as many carbohydrates, your insulin levels drop. This signals the kidneys to release sodium from your body. Losing approximately 10 pounds of water over a couple of days is not uncommon as water trails sodium out of your body. Glycogen is then transformed into glucose as the final energy source before switching to largely fatty acids.

Transitioning From Sugar to Fat for Energy

As your body switches from burning mainly sugar to fat for energy, your body will need to make some changes on the way. The number of side effects, if there are any, depend on your metabolic flexibility. Your body's metabolic flexibility is primarily its ability to metabolize different types of food. If you are used to eating a lot of carbohydrates and sugars, it can feel a lot like giving up other harmful substances like nicotine or alcohol, for example.

T3 Thyroid Hormone Levels May Decrease

T3 is a hormone produced by the thyroid that is associated with dietary carbohydrates. It plays a major role in the regulation of your body's temperature, metabolism, and heart rate.

Hormone Response and Rebalancing Cortisol

Cortisol takes on a lot of various roles in your body, including regulating blood sugar and controlling inflammation. During your transition, your body assumes that it is starving for sugar. This causes a release of cortisol to increase blood glucose. This is a natural stress response that we call "flight or fight" mode, which is the result of our ancestral instincts telling us to go hunt for food.

Purging Addictions

You may also encounter alterations in what Dr. Kevin Stock (2018) refers to as the "brain-body highway" that controls signaling between the gut and the brain. This communication highway impacts everything from hormones to neurotransmitters like dopamine, serotonin, and GABA, that play essential roles in your mood, cravings, and addictions. Similar to other substance addictions, you may experience withdrawal symptoms from foods or other substances (like sugar) to which you have become physically and neurologically addicted.

How to Deal With the Symptoms:

Be Prepared

By familiarizing yourself with potential symptoms, you are already taking a necessary step by comprehending and accepting the symptoms that may arise. After you have prepared yourself mentally, you can start preparing yourself physically. Keep in mind that these preparations will either completely prevent these symptoms or make them less sufferable. Everyone has different experiences because their body is unique in its functionality.

Eat Meat

Eat even more meat. Undereating is one of the main reasons why people go through adverse symptoms unnecessarily. It is normal to experience hunger early on in the process, but you should eat whenever you feel this way. You should not restrict macros or calories during the process because you could be missing out on essential nutrients.

Hydrate Efficiently

Measure your body weight and divide it by two. This is the minimum amount of water that you need to be drinking (in ounces) daily if you are experiencing any symptoms. After your body has fully adapted to the diet, you can start drinking to quench your thirst without measuring the amount of water you consume (as long as it is still a safe amount). Hydrating frequently is majorly important when you are adapting to new eating habits.

Electrolytes

You will lose a lot of excess water which means you will also lose a lot of electrolytes like sodium, potassium, magnesium, chloride, etc. Supplemental electrolytes can make a big difference in minimizing the effects that this can have on your body. Adding pure pink Himalayan rock salt to your food can provide extra sodium and chloride. This is helpful for those who struggle with sodium and chloride.

However, some people need help in the potassium and magnesium department as well.

There are a few ways to beat this shortage or loss like drinking meaty bone broth while continuing to consume water and sodium. This will add potassium to your diet which will stop some of the discomfort on a cellular level. It is crucial that the bones you use still have some meat on them because that is where the most potassium is stored. Using an ionic potassium supplement is also a popular solution among carnivores. It contains all the necessary electrolytes and nutrients that will ease your discomfort effectively. The recommended supplemental electrolyte daily ranges are K – 500-3,500 mg/day, Mg – 250-500 mg/day, and Na – 2-7g/day, according to Dr. Kevin Stock (2018).

Bowel Movement Problems

Gastrointestinal (GI) issues are very common, especially if you were previously following a low-fat diet. You might be ready to go full speed ahead, but your gallbladder may not be ready to handle a high amount of fat intake. You can reduce your fat intake by consuming leaner cuts of meat. This is not ideal, and it may be better to use some supplements for the next few weeks until the problem resolves.

You can begin with a simple lipase supplement that is preferably taken before meals. It will cause less frequent trips to the bathroom and ease your stomach. For most people, this helps quite a lot. If you are used to a very low-fat diet, your gallbladder may need some assistance until it is able to yield enough bile on its own. Taking ox bile with meals can work for this issue. Sometimes, not having a lot of stomach acid can be the problem and it is quite troublesome because it can result in GERD. A betaine HCl supplement can help with reflux and soothe some of the discomfort.

There are some cases where the type of fat consumed causes GI distress. If the supplements mentioned above are not helping, then your body might have some trouble digesting rendered fat. Rendered fat is cooked out of meat, becoming liquid. For example, if you prepare your food in a skillet, you might see fat start to liquify. This liquid fat can cause numerous problems if your body has a problem digesting it.

If this is the case, your bowel movements will change. Some people do not defecate as much as they used to. It is no cause for alarm, however, and it is extremely common, so this should not be treated as constipation. The amount or volume will also decrease which only means that your body digests and utilizes the meat more efficiently and, unlike before, there is less waste to get rid of.

Digestion and GI digestive issues, or at least changes, are nearly certain. Follow these steps to decrease discomfort if necessary:

It is recommended to take these supplements a few minutes before your meals.

- Lipase – 1-2 capsules (6,000-12,000 LU)

- Ox bile – 1-2 capsules (500-1,000 mg)

- Betaine HCl with pepsin – 1 capsule (500mg betaine HCl/20mg pepsin).

Problems with Sleep

According to Dr. Kevin Stock (2018), sleep is necessary to make us feel better overall, but insomnia is common during the first few weeks. The fact that you are heading to the bathroom more frequently can also disrupt your sleeping pattern. There are a few things that might help you to sleep better:

- Keep your room dark and cool. This way, your body will not be triggered by light or temperature during your sleep.

- Start getting ready for "sleep mode" two hours before bed. Switch off some electronics and let your mind and body know that it is time to rest. Get comfortable and try not to think or stress about anything work related or otherwise.

- Eat a few hours before bedtime and try to be aware of how much you are drinking in the afternoons and evenings, as this will result in fewer late night trips to the bathroom.

- Try your best to fall asleep before 11:00 p.m. as cortisol spikes occur more frequently if you stay up late.

- Sweating is a natural way to spruce up the detoxification system in your body. Since you will be feeding your body the nutrition it has been in need of, you can also give it the opportunity to drive out all of the toxins. You will help your body tremendously when you exercise and sweat frequently because it will not have to work as hard on the detoxification process. Please remember that your training performance will decrease a little bit for anywhere between one and six months, however, your ability to bounce back will be even stronger than before (Stock, 2018).

Chapter 4:

Transform Your Body and Your Mind

Weight Loss

Protein and Weight Loss

Your weight is dynamically controlled by your brain, specifically by an area of the brain called the hypothalamus. Your brain determines when and how much to eat by processing multiple types of information. The most vital signals sent to the brain are found in the form of hormones that alternate in response to feeding. When you consume more protein, your levels of satiety hormones GLP-1, peptide YY, and cholecystokinin increase. The hunger hormone ghrelin is then suppressed significantly, which obviously leads to less hunger. By reducing carbohydrates and replacing them with fat and protein, you can minimize the hunger hormone and increase the levels of various hormones that cause satiety. This entire process leads to minimal hunger throughout the day and is also one of the main reasons why protein can promote weight loss to a significant extent. You will realize that this satiated feeling becomes quite common once you settle into the carnivore diet (Gunnars, 2017).

Whenever you eat, some of the calories you consume are used to digest and metabolize the food. This is frequently called the thermic effect of food, or TEF for short. Despite the fact that not all researchers agree on the precise figures, it is argued that protein has a significantly higher thermic effect (20-30%), where carbohydrates (5-10%) and fat (0-3%) have much lower thermic effects. For example, the thermic effect of 30% for protein means that 100 calories of the protein amounts to only 70 usable calories. Because of the high thermic effect and several other factors, a high-level protein consumption will boost your metabolism. It enables your body to burn more calories throughout the day, and during sleep when your metabolism is considerably slower.

A high level of protein consumption has been proven to boost metabolism and the number of calories burned by about 80 to 100 per day. This effect is specifically noticeable during overfeeding, or while eating a caloric surplus. In one study, overfeeding with a high-protein diet increased calories burned by 260 per day. Due to the fact that they cause the burning of more calories, high-protein diets have a metabolic benefit over diets that are lower in protein. The more protein you eat, the more calories you burn.

Protein reduces hunger and appetite through numerous distinct structures. This can lead to an automatic reduction in calorie intake. Although the carnivore diet does not encourage calorie restricting, you will most likely consume fewer useless calories than before. This is because you will end up eating fewer calories without needing to count calories or deliberately control the size or number of portions.

Several studies have demonstrated that, when people boost their protein intake, they start eating less calories. This works on a meal-to-meal foundation, and results in a continuous day-to-day decrease in calorie intake as long as the protein intake is kept elevated. In one study, protein consumption at 30% of calories caused people to involuntarily drop their overall calorie intake by 441 calories per day, which is a massive amount. High-protein diets not only have a metabolic benefit, they also have an "appetite advantage," making it much simpler to cut calories in contrast with lower-protein diets. High-protein diets are very filling, so they lead to decreased hunger and appetite compared to lower-protein diets. This makes it simpler to limit calories on a high-protein diet (Gunnars, 2017).

Protein consumption causes weight loss without the efforts of conscious calorie restriction. Protein works on either end of the "calories in versus calories out" calculation. It lowers calories in and raises calories out. For this reason, it is not shocking to see high-protein diets resulting in weight loss, even without purposely restricting calories, portions, fat, or carbs.

A high-protein diet, such as the carnivore diet, promotes eating more protein and fewer or no carbohydrates to boost weight loss, improve energy, and enhance athletic performance. Protein is an indispensable nutrient for optimal health. It is accountable for a number of crucial functions in your body, including the behavior of hormones and enzymes, cell repair, and overall maintenance.

According to Very Well Fit (Frey, 2020), research suggests that a diet high in protein can help overweight and obese subjects lose more fat while preserving lean muscle mass. Diets like the carnivore diet that are high in protein, help to reduce hunger, boost satiety, improve metabolic rate, and maintain muscle mass. The carnivore diet is therefore one of the more successful diets or lifestyles to follow when you want to lose weight.

In general, a high-protein diet recommends getting more than 20% of your total calories from protein. That typically means eating fewer calories from carbohydrates or fats to keep your calories in balance (Frey, 2020). The carnivore diet, however, does not cap the amount of protein you consume daily because the end goal is to consume animal products only by the third level. Eating a diet that is high in protein provides numerous benefits, particularly when you are trying to lose weight.

Including protein in both your meals and snacks can help you to feel full and satisfied after you are finished eating. This satiated feeling will help you to eat and snack less throughout the day. As we now know, protein also helps you to develop and preserve muscle mass. The carnivore diet strengthens the body and a stronger body not only performs better generally throughout daily actions, but the muscles that are formed and maintained also burn more calories than fat, even at rest. When your meal is based on a few sources of protein, you will inevitably have less space on your plate for foods that are not recommended. Learning to eat different types of protein or meats may improve your diet as well. If you eat different cuts of beef, for example, you will not only benefit from the protein in the meat, but also from the healthy fat it provides.

In addition, you can burn a few extra calories when you eat animal products like meat because your body has to work harder to physically eat and digest the food. Scientists refer to this as the thermic effect of food (Frey, 2020). Surely, the number of calories that you burn in this instance is not necessarily a tremendous amount, but this is certainly a bonus, even if it does not affect your caloric intake significantly. Rather than focusing on calories or portion sizes, you should eat until you are full and try not to think about your next meal until you start getting hungry again.

A high-protein diet is an effective strategy for weight loss and the carnivore diet is especially so, because it encourages cutting out insignificant food groups, like fruits and grains. This concept has not been well received by everyone and some people might even argue that a more "well-rounded" diet is more effective. A lot of people tend to associate meat-heavy diets with weight gain and unhealthy cholesterol levels. It is not suggested that fruits and vegetables are the enemy, and they are still great foods to incorporate into your lifestyle, however, less is more in the carnivore diet. By minimizing the amount of carbs you consume, you also eliminate insulin spikes and without these spikes, your body is not triggered to store calories as body fat. People also successfully lose weight when switching to the carnivore diet, because it eliminates the need to snack and eat as often or as much as you would on a low-fat or high-carb diet. Hunger and cravings are the main culprits of weight gain which makes the carnivore lifestyle ideal for those who struggle with these issues.

Reduced Inflammation

One animal product, except for the essential meat products, that can improve your health tremendously is bone broth. In fact, it is quite essential that you incorporate it in your meal plan. There is also evidence that shows that gelatinous proteins like bone broth can improve cartilage health among other things.

Bone broth is made by boiling the bones and connective tissue of animals. It is a highly nutritious stock that is commonly used in soups, sauces, and gravies. It has also recently become popular as a health drink and supplement. It is also another food source that our ancestors used, and it dates back to prehistoric times when hunter-gatherers turned unpalatable animal parts like bones, hooves, and knuckles into a liquid substance that they could consume easily for extra nutrients. It can be made by using the bones from almost any animal. The most popular broths usually come from beef, pork, lamb, and chicken. Marrow and connective tissues like feet, hooves, beaks, and gizzards can also be used (McDonell, 2020).

McDonell (2020) also states that animal bones are filled with calcium, magnesium, potassium, phosphorus, and other trace minerals. These are the minerals needed to build and strengthen your own bones. Connective tissue provides you with glucosamine and chondroitin, natural compounds found in cartilage that are known to support joint health. Marrow also provides vitamin A, vitamin K2, minerals like zinc, iron, boron, manganese, and selenium, as well as omega-3 and omega-6 fatty acids. All these animal parts also contain the protein collagen, which turns into gelatin when cooked and yields several important amino acids.

The amino acids found in bone broth, including glycine and arginine, have strong anti-inflammatory properties. Arginine may be especially useful for combating chronic inflammation. One animal study shows that dispensing oral arginine to mice with asthma reduced airway inflammation and improved symptoms of asthma. Another study in rats indicates that supplementing with arginine could help fight inflammation in people struggling with obesity

(McDonell, 2020). Although some inflammation is necessary, chronic inflammation can lead to several serious illnesses and diseases like heart disease, diabetes, metabolic syndrome, Alzheimer's disease, arthritis, and many different types of cancer.

High fat, low-carbohydrate diets, like the carnivore or keto diet, have become popular tools for weight management. High fat and low-carb diets have proven to be beneficial for weight-loss, cardiovascular risk factors, and inflammation in people with obesity. In a study (Ruth et al., 2013, p. 1780) where obese subjects (29.0–44.6 kg/m2) were recruited from Boston Medical Center and put on a hypocaloric LFHC (n=26) or HFLC (n=29) diet for 12 weeks it showed that a high-fat low-carb diet showed greater improvements in blood lipids and systemic inflammation as well as weight-loss. The small-scale study also shows that high-fat low-carb diets may be more beneficial to cardiovascular health and inflammation in obese adults compared to low-fat/high-carb diets.

The study (Ruth et al., 2013, p. 1780) was done on subjects aged 21-62 years. As a percentage of daily calories, the HFLC group consumed 33.5% protein, 56.0% fat, and 9.6% carbohydrates and the LFHC group consumed 22.0% protein, 25.0% fat, and 55.7% carbohydrates. There were notable changes in the percentage of body weight, lean and fat mass, blood pressure, flow-mediated dilation, hip-waist ratio, hemoglobin A1C, fasting insulin, and glucose. Glucose and insulin response to a 2-hour oral glucose tolerance test did not differ.

Improved Heart Health

In a recent Norwegian diet involvement study (FATFUNC) published in The American Journal of Clinical Nutrition, study leader assistant Prof. Simon Nitter Dankel and colleagues have doubted and reversed the dietary theory that saturated fat is unhealthy for most people. This theory has eclipsed health literature for more than 50 years. The idea of restricting saturated fats to support a healthy body weight and reduce the risk of chronic disease has been widely received and welcomed in health guidelines for years, even decades (Nichols, 2016). Lately however, scientists and health organizations have held conflicting views on the threats of saturated fats.

The American Heart Association (AHA) agrees with the government's warnings and reiterates that the intake of saturated fats can enable higher levels of "bad" cholesterol in the blood that might raise the risk of heart disease. The Academy of Nutrition and Dietetics, however, recommends de-stressing the position of saturated fat in developing heart disease, due to the absence of evidence connecting the two. Most foods that are innately rich in saturated fat come from animal sources, comprising meat and dairy products. The AHA suggests restricting saturated fats, such as those found in butter, cheese, red meat, and other animal-based foods, based on years of sensible science, they say. Dankel and his team examined the risk of saturated fat on 38 men with obesity. The partakers were divided into two groups and followed either a very high fat/low-carbohydrate diet, or a low-fat/high-carbohydrate diet for 12 weeks. The researchers measured fat mass in the abdominal region, liver, and heart. They also assessed cardiovascular risk factors (Nichols, 2016).

The present theory regarding saturated fat would indicate that the high-fat/low-carbohydrate group would be at greater risk of heart disease than the low-fat/high-carbohydrate group. Although, this was not the case, there was no difference between the groups. According to Otter Nygard, a professor and cardiologist involved in the study (Nichols, 2016), the very high intake of total and saturated fat did not raise the estimated risk of cardiovascular diseases provided to the study. He also added that subjects who were on the very high-fat diet also had significant improvements in several important cardiometabolic risk factors, such as ectopic fat storage, blood pressure, blood lipids (triglycerides), insulin, and blood sugar.

Ph.D. candidate, Vivian Veum (Nichols, 2016), also stated that they looked at effects of total and saturated fat in the context of a healthy diet rich in fresh, low processed, and nutritious foods, including high amounts of vegetables and rice instead of flour-based products. He also mentions that the primary fat sources were also low-processed products, mainly butter, cream, and cold-pressed oils. The intake of energy, proteins, polyunsaturated fatty acids, and food types was comparable across both groups, the only difference was that the quantity and the consumption of added sugar was kept to a minimum.

The energy intake of both groups was mostly within the normal range. Those participants that increased their energy intake still saw a reduction in fat stores and risk of disease.

Ph.D. candidate, Johnny Laupsa-Borge (Nichols, 2016), adds that their findings indicate that the overriding principle of a healthy diet is not in the quantity of fat or carbohydrates, but in the quality of the foods we eat. The FATFUNC study disputes the theory that the path to heart disease from saturated fat is paved by raising levels of "bad" low-density lipoprotein (LDL) cholesterol in the blood. The study not only observed no significant rise in LDL cholesterol, but they also found that the high-fat diet was only linked to an increase in "good" cholesterol levels. Nygård (Nichols 2016) once again adds that the results indicate that most healthy people likely endure a high consumption of saturated fat well, as long as the fat quality is good and total energy intake is not too high. It may even be healthful, which falls in the same range as the carnivore diet. Dankel (Nichols, 2016) concludes that the alleged health risks of eating good-quality fats have been greatly overstated. It may be more critical for public health to promote cutbacks in processed flour-based products, highly processed fats, and foods with added sugar.

Higher Testosterone in Men

According to Dr. James Elist (Elist, 2017), amino acid chains that relate to peptide bonds are responsible for forming a protein molecule. Diverse proteins have different lengths of amino acid chains. A complete protein will contain all vital amino acids. For instance, some examples of healthy protein sources are eggs, dairy, and meat.

Testosterone production and muscle mass increase significantly depends on the total consumption of protein and the type of protein used. Inadequate protein consumption can decrease muscle mass and lower testosterone production. For maximum muscle gain, a person requires 0.8 grams of protein per pound of lean mass. In fact, 0.37 grams per pound is sufficient to maintain the positive nitrogen balance in habituated body builders.

Studies found that a high-fat/low-fiber diet does indeed increase testosterone. Researchers created a controlled study of 43 men, half of whom ate the high-fat/low-fiber diet and the other half ate a low-fat/high-fiber diet. The group that ate the high-fat/low-fiber diet had a 13% increase in testosterone (Dorgan et al., 1996, p. 853).

They conducted a measured feeding study to calculate the effects of fat and fiber consumption on plasma and urine sex hormones (like testosterone) in men. The study had a crossover layout and involved 43 healthy men aged 19-56 years. The men were originally randomly assigned to either a low-fat/high-fiber or high-fat/low-fiber diet for 10 weeks and after a two-week phasing out period, they had to cross over to the other diet. The energy content of the diets was varied to maintain constant body weight, but averaged approximately 3170 kcal per day on both diets. The low-fat diet provided 18.8% of energy from fat with a ratio of polyunsaturated to saturated fat (P:S) of 1.3, whereas the high-fat diet provided 41.0% of energy from fat with a P:S of 0.6 (Dorgan et al., 1996, p. 853).

Overall dietary fiber intake from the low- and high-fat diets averaged 4.6 and 2.0 g MJ-1.d-1, respectively. This means that the plasma concentrations overall and sex-hormone-binding-globulin (SHBG)-bound testosterone were 13% and 15% higher independently, on the high-fat/low-fiber diet and the dissimilarity from the low-fat/high-fiber diet was notable for the SHBG-bound fraction (P = 0.04). The male's daily urinary flow of testosterone was also 13% higher with the high-fat/low-fiber diet than with the low-fat/high-fiber diet (P = 0.01). Equivalently, their urinary ejection of estradiol and estrone and their 2-hydroxy metabolites were 12-28% lower with the high-fat/low-fiber diet (P < or = 0.01). Results of this study suggest that diet may alter endogenous sex hormone metabolism in men (Dorgan et al., 1996, p. 853).

Increased Mental Clarity, Improved Memory, and Focus

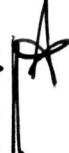

Meat and animal products are considered brain-healthy foods, as they promote better mood stability, stronger focus, and more energy. People who suffer from concentration issues also report less distractibility, less tiredness in the late morning and mid-afternoon, and fewer cravings for sugary substances when they are on a high-protein eating plan. Protein helps balance blood sugar and focus and gives the necessary building blocks for brain health especially. Great sources of protein include eggs, dairy, red meats, and bone broth. Protein powders can also be a good source of protein; however, the ingredients label should be studied efficiently to make sure the product is not high in sugar or other possible toxins. Starting and ending each day with protein will boost your focus, concentration skills, and memory (Amen, 2020). Our brains are dependent on protein to function and we need to consume it frequently because it cannot be produced on its own. When you keep your protein intake at a higher level, your brain is able to make use of all that energy to work at its best capacity.

According to Hyson (2020), similar to the ketogenic diet, carnivore dieters account that they experience clearer thoughts and have better focus shortly after starting the carnivore diet. Also similar to the ketogenic diet, is the break-in or adjustment period where your body has to learn how to fuel and nourish your system without carbs, so you will probably feel lethargic and moody at first. You may also have some issues with your sleeping pattern and even experience bad breath, which is an early indication that your body is producing ketones, but you can ride it out. As we already know from previous chapters, within a few days or a week, you will feel sharper than ever, possibly even better than if you were doing a basic level ketogenic diet.

According to Munsey (Hyson, 2020), your whole system snaps into place after approximately two weeks.

Improved Mood and Emotional Stability

It is no secret that our diets can contribute to our emotional capacity and as you read earlier, your diet can have an immense impact on your mental health. There is proof that indicates a link between diet and depression, and a role for dietary modification in treating depression. It is progressively clear that there is a solid connection between gut health and depression, thanks to the gut-brain axis. Many professionals also consider systemic inflammation to be a root cause of depression. Systemic inflammation is also said to respond well to the carnivore diet. Consequently, any diet that expands gut health and lowers inflammation is potentially beneficial. Psychiatrist, Dr. Georgia Ede, has become an honest advocate of the carnivore lifestyle for depression, as well as other mental health disorders, due to these findings. She also accurately points out that the brain needs fat, including cholesterol, and other nutrients that are much more plentiful in animal foods than in plant foods, such as choline, carnitine, Omega-3 fatty acids EPA and DHA, and vitamin B12. A 2015 review of dietary interferences for depression and anxiety found that they often include commendations to reduce red meat consumption, but that makes them less likely to be operative. Similarly, one study found women who eat less red meat were at larger risk for major depression (Sisson, 2020).

Non-pharmacological methods for the treatment of depression and anxiety are of growing importance, with promising evidence strengthening a role for lifestyle reasons in the development of these disorders. Data-based evidence confirms a relationship between habitual diet quality and depression. There is not much known about the contributory effects of diet on mental health outcomes. Consequently, a systematic review was undertaken of randomized regulated and inspected trials of dietary intercession that used depression and/or anxiety results and aimed to identify qualities of program success. Of the 1,274 articles found, 17 met suitability criteria and were included. All of them stated depression outcomes and 10 stated anxiety or total mood disturbance. Compared with a control condition, almost half (47%) of the studies detected substantial effects on depression scores in favor of the treatment group. The outstanding studies reported a null effect. Effective dietary intercessions were based on a single delivery mode, recruited a dietitian and were less likely to recommend lower red meat intake, choose leaner meat products or follow a low-cholesterol diet (Opie et al., 2015, p. 2079).

Since 2009, there has been growing evidence of a link between habitual diet quality and depression and anxiety. In two of these studies, it is reported that women with higher scores on a dietary pattern characterized by beef and other traditional foods were less prone to have anxiety, major depressive dysthymia, or bipolar disorders. The fact that red meat was a prominent component of this protective dietary pattern was of some importance, as earlier studies analyzing dietary patterns as forecasters of illness have detected red meat to be a part of damaging dietary patterns. Furthermore, there are published studies from Australia and Scandinavia stating that vegetarians and/or people who do not consume a lot of meat have poorer mental health than those who customarily eat meat, although the direction of the relationship between vegetarian status and mental health is unclear (Jacka et al., 2012, p. 196).

Chapter 5:

Recipes for Success

This chapter will provide you with a variety of recipes that you can use while following the carnivore diet. Since this diet is largely based on intuitive eating, and does not require you to eat a set amount of meals, these can be eaten for breakfast, lunch or dinner, based on your own schedule and preferences.

How Often Do I Need to Eat on This Diet?

When you start considering the carnivore diet, you will start noticing luxuriously packaged, lustrous-colored foods that were not a part of our Paleolithic existence at all. Except for the fact that our ancestors did not consume processed junk foods and candies at all and our hunter-gatherer ancestors did not have those options, it is also important to note that these foods are not the only unnatural outcome of our modern lifestyles. Sleep disturbance and travel was also not a big thing during those times as it is now and our ancestors did not have the means to move between time zones. This briefly explains why we experience problems with sleep and why our bodies often suffer when we travel.

The human body is mainly driven by circadian rhythms that predict when we should be awake or active, resting or asleep, and even what and when we eat. Modern technology and changes such as electricity and convenience-based foods disturb these rhythms and place evolutionary stress on our bodies. Without realizing it, we become influenced by these concepts and it affects our diet and overall health to a great extent. This theory is presented to us by a recent review published in the Proceedings of the National Academy of Science by Dr. Mark Mattson et al. They concluded that our health is not solely based on what we eat, but largely also by when we eat and how we have disrupted our circadian rhythms (Connor, 2014).

Natural 24-hour rhythms pervade the entire animal and even the vegetable kingdoms. In humans, circadian alterations have been found in over 10% of our articulated genes influencing almost all of our bodies' metabolic, neurological, and endocrine pathways. The suprachiasmatic nucleus (SCN) in the hypothalamus acts as our "master clock," responding to daily light-dark cycles through photoreceptive ganglion cells in our retinas. Mattson et al. questioned whether the invention of artificial light and shift work disturbed this circadian clock, promoting longer daily cycles of consumption (Connor, 2014).

This means that, due to our inability to function without electricity, screens, lights, and other modern disturbances, we have disrupted the communication patterns between our eyes and our brains and it has become difficult for our bodies to enter a stage where we can distinguish between day and night. Obviously, we can tell whether it is night or day, but our circadian rhythms are gravely disturbed by this and that is why we are still active and eating during the night.

Sequentially, our inconsistent eating habits affect our biological clocks. Two of the main routes in our bodies that react to fasting and feeding—cAMP response element binding protein (CREB) for fasting and the insulin-dependent mammalian target of rapamycin (MTOR) for feeding—can directly impact circadian alterations. In one mouse study, researchers were able to use feeding to rapidly shift liver oscillations 10 hours out of sync with the light-sensitive SCN.6 (Connor, 2014). This disruptive and intrusive cycle of reformed eating habits and disturbed rhythms that are constantly feeding off each other is most likely the major cause of obesity and metabolic problems.

This cycle of altered eating behavior and unsettled rhythms building upon one another may be a major cause of obesity and metabolic disorders. Our natural eating patterns have been disrupted and our normal consumption methods are not a means of unhealthy or healthy lifestyles, but more a consequence of unbalanced circadian rhythms.

Recent reports (Connor, 2014) of hunter-gatherer eating behavior and Dr. Cordain's own ethnographic research, describe a very different eating cycle. Hunter-gatherers were more susceptible to consuming a single large meal in the late afternoon or evening after spending the day hunting and gathering on little to no food. Hunter-gatherers did not eat consistently day to day. While anthropological research has deflated the idea of intermittent starvation in Paleolithic times, without the modern need for a stocked fridge and preservative-packed foods, hunter-gatherers likely had frequent days of extremely reduced energy intake.

The health benefits of a calorie restricted diet, also regarding a positive effect on seniority, have already been determined. In their review, Mattson et al. go a step further by initiating two timing-dependent variations on a CR diet that are more common with Paleolithic behavior and may actually elevate the health benefits. There are two eating patterns that were concluded. These include a time-restricted feeding (TRF) diet where any form of eating/drinking is limited to a brief time period during the day (a four- to eight-hour window) to mimic life before modern electricity and technologies, and the second, an intermittent energy restriction consisting of periodic days where calories are greatly reduced (i.e., just 500 calories) such as twice per week, an eating pattern that would be more consistent with a Paleolithic lifestyle (Connor, 2014).

So how does the carnivore diet play into this research? Well the carnivore diet is not a calorie-restricted diet, but it does encourage the notion that you should only eat when you are hungry and stop eating once you are full. Our ancestors did not count their calories, nor did they time their eating schedules. They ate instinctively. In other words, they ate when they were hungry, if they could find food. When you are living the carnivore lifestyle, you will likely notice that you are not as hungry anymore. This is because the fat and protein that are found in animal-based foods keep you fuller longer so that you can use energy as your body requires. It is loosely based on the idea that, just like our Paleolithic ancestors, we should eat to fuel our bodies and not to indulge. Surely, this does not mean that you are not allowed to enjoy or like your food. It just means that it works to your advantage to eat during the day and not at night, and if you can, you should try eating two main meals a day and avoid snacking, although adjusting to this way of eating can take a long time.

How sleep influences appetite is one popular theory about the relation between weight and sleep. While we sometimes think of appetite as simply a matter of a grumbling in the stomach, neurotransmitters, which are chemical messengers that enable neurons (nerve cells) to communicate with each other, actually regulate it. It is known that the neurotransmitters ghrelin and leptin are central to appetite. Hunger is promoted by ghrelin, and leptin leads to feeling full. Throughout the day, the body gradually raises and lowers the levels of these neurotransmitters, suggesting the need to eat calories. A lack of sleep may influence the control of these neurotransmitters by the body. In one study, relative to those who got 10 hours of sleep, men who got 4 hours of sleep had increased ghrelin and decreased leptin (Truong, 2020).

In individuals who are sleep deprived, this dysregulation of ghrelin and leptin may contribute to increased appetite and decreased feelings of fullness. In addition, several studies have also shown that sleep deprivation affects food preferences. Individuals who are sleep-deprived prefer to select diets rich in calories and carbohydrates. The body's endocannabinoid system and orexin, a neurotransmitter targeted by certain sleep aids, are other theories about the connection between sleep and increased appetite. Many researchers believe that the relationship between sleep and neurotransmitter dysregulation is complicated and more studies are needed to further understand the neurobiological relationship (Truong, 2020).

Metabolism is a chemical mechanism in which the body absorbs the energy required to live on what we consume and drink. Our metabolisms are a part of all of our collective practices, from breathing to exercise, and everything in between. Although activities like exercise can increase metabolism temporarily, sleep cannot. In fact, metabolism slows down during sleep by about 15%, hitting its lowest level in the morning (Truong, 2020). Seeing that our metabolisms are slower in the morning, it might be a good idea to avoid skipping breakfast in order to give your metabolism that boost or kick starter that it needs. Sleep is extremely important when you are on the carnivore diet, especially at the beginning.

As your body adjusts to lower carbohydrate intake, you will also start to feel fatigued. Although these side effects, like fatigue and lethargy, tend to subside shortly after the first two weeks, you will still want to focus on improving your sleeping patterns. Napping during the day could disrupt your sleep cycle, so try to stick it out. If you feel like you struggle to fall asleep at night, try going lights out and screens off by a certain time. This will give your brain an instinctive hint that it is time for bed. You can also cut back on caffeinated drinks by 4:00 in the afternoon, or even earlier, as caffeine prevents your brain from winding down. Another way to have some decent shut eye is to make sure that your room is cool and well ventilated. You will feel less inclined to wake up if you are as comfortable as possible, and some people even purchase weighted blankets or sheets to cozy up during bedtime.

You will also notice how sleep impacts your mental health and clarity. People who do not get enough sleep, too much sleep, or sleep during strange hours of the day tend to struggle more mentally. Your mental health and sleeping patterns go hand in hand. If you are anxious, you will sleep less, and if you are depressed, you will likely sleep more. Make sure that you check on yourself mentally and physically before, during, and after the process. Mental health is equally important as physical health and if your mind is not healthy, your body will follow suit. It can be quite difficult to deal with monitoring your health and changing your eating habits at the same time; however, it is important to remember that the amount of protein and fat that you will be consuming will certainly fuel your mind as well as your body and it will improve naturally.

Alternatively, as you adjust to these new eating patterns, you will find the balance of meals that works best for you and your body. Some people only eat lunch and dinner, while others use intermittent fasting in addition to the carnivore diet requirements. The ketogenic diet follows many of the same tenets as the carnivore diet, and most keto recipes can be easily adapted to fit this plan. The key is making sure that each meal/snack is high in protein and fats, and that you eat until you are totally full and satisfied in order to avoid unnecessary snacking or to curb some of those annoying cravings. Steak for breakfast? No problem!

A Complete Guide to Pork and Beef Cuts

Once you start your carnivore journey you will realize how important it is to know the difference between different cuts of meat. It can be convenient and beneficial to know which part of the animal you are using and how to prepare it properly. The most prevalent cuts are found in pork and beef. The goal of this section is to provide you with sufficient knowledge of the different cuts and to give you some tips on how you can improve your cooking skills. You might even find which cuts work better for you and learn a bit more about the art of shopping for a carnivore diet. Remember to check the color, texture, and overall appearance of the meat. It is also quite important to seek out organic options instead of mass produced types of meat.

Some cuts, like Pork belly for example, are not actually the stomach. It is mostly the meat that sits around the tummy and it is a reasonably sized cut. It is an easy one to prepare because you can add a few spices and braise it, roast it, or add it to a pressure cooker.

Pork Loin Chops

Pork chops is a term used to describe various cuts. It is a generic term but the most popular cuts that are referred to as pork chops are loin chops, rib chops, top loin chops, or pork shoulder chops. They are extremely delicious and rather easy to prepare. They can easily be cooked on the grill or even on the stove with a pan or skillet. Pork loin chops usually have T-shaped bone which is easy to spot. The chops that come from the rib on the other hand have a thinner and often longer bone attached to it. The top loin chops are more likely packaged in the form of fillets and are deboned. They are also rounder in shape but still as easy to prepare and equally delicious. Shoulder chops, also known as blade chops, are a little less tender and need some more attention. They are better suited for slow-cooking and often require some type of marinade to make them less tough. In this case, tenderizing might be a good idea.

Pork Crown Roast

You will be able to seek this one out quite easily. It is a rack of trimmed meat that is tied together to form a circle, this is why it is called a crown roast. It will most likely exist of two racks. The middle part of the crown can be filled with different ingredients like herbs, spices, or other condiments that liven up the dish.

Pork Cutlets

Pork cutlets are deboned and have a similar cut as a beef sirloin steak would. It is quite thin and often rounded. It is usually a leaner type of pork cut that is quick and easy to prepare. They can be braised or slow-cooked however it will cause the meat to break apart quite quickly, so the grill or pan might be a better option for this particular cut. It is also a great alternative to a beef patty and is often used to make pork sandwiches or pulled-pork.

Ham

Ham is derived from the leg of the pig, mostly from the top part because the part of the leg downwards is referred to as the shank. They are usually smoked or cured beforehand, but they can also be bought fresh. It is important to know how this cut is prepared before adding it to your carnivore menu because it can often be overprocessed. Purchasing smoked ham is better suited to the carnivore diet than the other options.

Pork Loin

The parts that are referred to as the loin are usually cut from the shoulder, rump, or centre. They are also known as tenderloins or loin chops. The cuts that come from the shoulder are fattier. The rump is bonier, but still as tender and the cuts that are derived from the centre are leaner. They are also often found in the form of a roast that is tied with string. These cuts are quite popular because they are tender and a little pricey. However, they are easily paired with other side dishes and totally worth it.

Pork Ribs

The back ribs, also known as baby back ribs, are small and hearty. They are meaty and small which makes them easier to eat. Hence the nickname "baby back ribs." They can be deliciously prepared on the grill or even popped in the oven. Their convenience-factor and size is arguably what makes them so popular. There are also country-style ribs and spareribs. Both are tasty and packed with flavor. Country-style ribs can be identified by the amount of fat attached to the cut because they are the fattier option where spareribs have less meat and fat attached, which makes them a leaner option. Country-style ribs are often deboned and can also be used as a delicious topping for a low-carb pizza topping. Spareribs are not as meaty and can therefore be added to stews, soups, and used to make bone broth. Do not let the fact that they are not as fatty or meaty stop you from trying them out.

Pork Roasts

There is a whole list of cuts that can be purchased as roasts. They are usually identifiable by their ability to be baked in the oven. Pork blade roasts are rather common and inexpensive, which explains their popularity among carnivores. They have a high fat content and are packed with flavor. If they still contain some bones, you can easily remove them yourself or ask your butcher to debone it for you. You can also purchase centre loin roasts that are deboned to make a delicious roast with some added fat.

Pork Sausages

Pork sausages are the most common forms of sausage that you will find. It is advised to purchase fresh pork sausages and not the ones that are already cooked or cured. When you do purchase pre-cooked sausages, make sure they are smoked instead of cooked, cured, or processed. As a carnivore, you should be careful about consuming processed sausages, as they could be high in preservatives that hold no nutritional value. Pork sausages are easy to prepare and work well on the grill or in a pan. They can often be prepared without seasoning or other condiments because they hold a lot of flavor.

Pork Hocks and Shanks

These cuts are usually taken from the shins of the pig and they can also be purchased smoked. They go well with stews and soups and can be used to make bone broth, which is an essential product in the carnivore for its nutritional value. If the skin is removed, the cuts will be called shanks, usually sold raw, and will respond very well to braising (Watson, 2020).

Pork Butt and Shoulder

Pork shoulder cuts come from a thicker section of the shoulder that has intense marbling and also the pork blade which is the triangular section that would be attached to the buttocks. Both of these cuts require slower cooking methods like barbecuing, braising, or stewing. They are quite versatile when they are cooked longer, but not suitable for grilling or frying.

Pork Back Fat

This is the hard fat largely cut from the back of the pig. It is not the same as the fat that comes from the belly because it is not as soft. It needs to be ground or processed in order to make it usable. It is usually found in sausages and you can easily spot it by looking for the white bits of fat mixed with the meat inside of a sausage casing. It prevents the sausage stuffing from becoming too dry and adds some fattiness to the sausage itself. It also contains a substantial amount of moisture which makes the sausage tender and juicy.

Pork Lard

Lard is mostly used as a substitute for cooking oil and it is rendered fat taken from the meat. It adds a lot of flavor to any meal and is made from softer fat than pork back fat. It does not have a particular taste and it will merely fatten up your dish without altering the taste in any sense. The fat is usually derived from the surrounding parts of the kidneys or loins.

Beef

There are many different cuts of beef that you can use to make the most of your carnivore journey. Humans mainly consume the primal cuts of the animal because they are known as the most resourceful and consumable parts which include the loin, flank, chuck, sirloin, brisket and more. They can also be further categorized into sub-primal cuts. (Midhani, 2018).

Loin, Short Loin, Strip Loin Cuts

The loin, short loin, and strip loin cuts are well known for being some of the leaner cuts of beef that you will find. They work well with high heat and are great for the grill, pan, and oven. When you are purchasing these cuts, you can search for T-bone, porterhouse, or tenderloin beef steaks. They are best suited for dry heat, which means that no cooking oil or added fat is necessary because the meat needs to be in direct contact with the heat source through the grill, pan, or oven dish surface.

Sirloin Cuts

The sirloin cuts, like filet mignon or beef strips, come from the parts of the animal that are closer to the rear.

The same principles as for other loin cuts apply to these as well. They are especially good for fast cooking dishes like stir fry, as they tend to become too soft when they are slowly cooked or boiled. For the best outcome, avoid any pressure or slow cooking methods.

Rib Cuts

Rib cuts in general have a higher fat content overall and some of the cuts are well suited for slower cooking methods and even roasting. However, cuts like rib eye steaks do not do well with slow cooking and will be more fitting to prepare in the pan or on the grill. This could be because the rib eye steaks are a bit more on the tender side and they tend to soften up quite easily compared to other rib cuts.

Chuck Cuts

This is where slow cooking starts to come into play with some good cuts for pot roasts. These cuts are more commonly known as blade cuts, chuck eye, or country-style ribs However, you will also find lots of chuck cuts that are good for grilling like top blade, ranch steak, and/or shoulder steak. Out of all of these sections, chuck is the one with the most variety, as there is a cut for every style of cooking. Chuck is also considerably inexpensive and can be utilized to a great extent throughout your carnivore journey.

Brisket Cuts

It is really hard to mess up a good brisket, and it does not matter which cut you choose. Whether it is a flat or point cut, they both need to be slow cooked. For most people, brisket point works better than brisket flat, because the flat cut is a bit leaner. Be careful when you decide to slow cook a brisket. It is a reasonably forgiving piece of meat, but the line between deliciously tender and juicy versus chewy and dry is rather thin.

Round Cuts

When it comes to round cuts, it is best to divide them into the two parts that are both derived from the back legs. The top parts work well with high heat and dry heat cooking while the bottom, rump, and eye roasts prefer slower cooking methods or oven roasting. These cuts are generally thicker, with a lower fat content and require some extra attention while being prepared. It is advised to do a little bit of research before you attempt to add these to your menu plan. However, beef is relatively easy to prepare overall, so there is no need to feel intimidated.

Plate and Flank Cuts

In this case, only the short ribs should be slow cooked; the flank and skirt steak will taste their best grilled or pan fried on high heat. Luckily, there are a lot of recipes with solid instructions that can make the cooking process less tedious.

Other Cuts

Beef cuts come in all shapes and sizes, so it is almost impossible to name each one individually. 'Other' refers to anything that does not fall into the same categories as the main cuts and portions. You can find stewing steak cuts, beef burgers, corned beef, as well as minced or ground beef in this category. Shanks are from the legs of the cow, and are arguably one of the most exciting beef cuts available that are also perfect for slow cooking. Another underrated cut of beef is the cheek. Beef cheeks are often discarded and not the most popular cut of beef. However, a lot of top restaurants have it on their menus and it should be considered when you start planning your own meals. It is also one of the most nutritious and convenient cuts to be slow cooked. This beef cut will spruce up your pot roast by making it better than ever before (Midhani, 2018).

Meals

Carnivore Flapjack Patties

These carnivore flapjack style patties can be perfect for breakfast, as a snack, or for dinner.

Time: 30-40 minutes

Serving Size: 10 servings

Prep Time: 10 minutes

Cook Time: 20-30 minutes

Nutritional Facts/Info: (Per Serving)

Calories: 592.0

Carbs: 0.9 g

Fat: 38.7 g

Protein: 60.2 g

Ingredients:
- 6 oz pork sausage
- 2 eggs
- 2 oz pork rinds

Directions:

1. Preheat the oven to 375°F and prepare a baking pan with foil and non-stick cooking spray.
2. Using a blender or food processor, crush the pork rinds into a fine flour-like substance.
3. Combine the eggs and the sausage in a mixing bowl and then stir in the pork rinds.
4. Form into thin rounded shapes on the greased baking pan.
5. Bake for 20-30 minutes depending on the thickness of your patties.
6. Allow the patties to cool once they are finished before removing them from the pan.

Carnivore Breakfast Stack

This breakfast stack is filled with carnivorous nourishment and guaranteed to keep you satisfied. Dairy-free? Just forget the cheese. Not wanting to be quite this plant-free? Add in some slices of ripe avocado or tomato.

Time: 10 minutes

Serving Size: 1 serving

Prep Time: 5 minutes

Cook Time: 5 minutes

Nutritional Facts/Info:

Calories: 448

Carbs: 1 g

Fat: 36 g

Protein: 33 g

Ingredients:
- 2 beef patties
- 1 egg
- 1 oz cheddar cheese
- 1 tsp butter (unsalted)

Directions:
1. In any large skillet, melt the butter over medium-high heat. Once the butter is melted, cook the patties until they are brown on the side, then flip them over and cook for another 2-3 minutes, or until they are cooked through.
2. Using the same pan, start frying your egg. Add additional butter if the pan is not greased enough. Try not to overcook the egg to prevent a dry breakfast, although it is up to you and your specific preferences.
3. To assemble the stack, place one patty on a plate, then top it with the fried egg, slice of

cheese, and the other patty. If you want to add avocado and tomato, be sure to stack it on top of the cheese for the best results.

Bacon and Chuck Stew

Stews make great hearty meals that can be rather easy to prepare. You can add the veggies if you would like to, or opt for the meat only.

Time: 7 hours 10 minutes

Serving Size: 8 servings

Prep Time: 10 minutes

Cook Time: 7 hours

Nutritional Facts/Info:

Calories: 594.4

Carbs: 5.1 g

Fat: 38.5 g

Protein: 52 g

Ingredients:
- 1 pack uncured bacon

- 2-3 lb beef chuck (arm pot roast)
- 2 large onions (raw)
- 2 cups cabbage (shredded)
- 1 garlic clove
- 3 tsp sea salt
- 1 tsp thyme (fresh)
- 2 cups beef bone broth

Directions:

1. Turn on your slow cooker and put it on low, add the ingredients in the following order:
2. Bacon slices to cover the bottom, onion slices and garlic, beef chuck, cabbage, thyme, and finally the broth.
3. Sprinkle a few pinches of sea salt and a decent amount of freshly ground black pepper.
4. Cook the stew on low for 7 hours.
5. Serve warm for the best results.

Meaty Quiche

Everyone loves a nice quiche, whether for breakfast, a snack, or during teatime. This meaty quiche recipe is carnivore-friendly and easier than you might expect. It is also a subtle way to incorporate something meaty into a social event like a brunch or party. For extra protein, you can add some extra meaty bits like chicken or beef.

Time: 55 minutes

Serving Size: 8 servings

Prep Time: 5 minutes

Cook Time: 50 minutes

Nutritional Facts/Info:

Calories: 257.5

Carbs: 1.2 g

Fat: 21.2 g

Protein: 16.3 g

Ingredients:
- 8 oz sausage and bacon crumbles
- 6 oz spiral sliced ham (chopped)
- 4 oz Swiss cheese (shredded)
- 4 oz cheddar cheese (shredded)
- 3 eggs
- 3 egg whites
- ½ cup heavy whipping cream
- ½ cup almond milk - coconut almond blend (unsweetened)
- ½ tsp salt
- ¼ tsp black pepper
- ¼ tsp onion powder

Directions:

1. Preheat the oven to 350°F.
2. Grease a round casserole dish with cooking spray or unsalted butter.
3. Place all of the meat products in the casserole dish. If you decide to grease the casserole dish with butter, make sure that the butter is evenly distributed and melted before you add the meat.
4. Sprinkle the cheese on top of the meat.
5. Whisk the eggs, egg whites, cream, milk, and seasonings together.
6. Carefully pour the egg mixture over the meat and cheese.
7. Bake the quiche mixture in the preheat oven for 35-45 minutes or until it is slightly golden and well set.
8. Let it rest for 10 minutes before slicing. If you can, let it cool down completely in order to keep it from falling apart.

Soupy Steak Stew

If you have some leftover steak and bones and don't know what to do with them, this recipe is the answer. You can also use fresh steak and bones; whatever floats your gravy boat.

Time: 2 hours 40 minutes

Serving Size: serves 6

Prep Time: 10 minutes

Cook Time: 2 hours 30 minutes

Nutritional Facts/Info:

Calories: 419.0

Carbs: 31.9 g

Fat: 10.2 g

Protein: 33.1 g

Ingredients:

- leftover or fresh steak and bones
- sea salt
- water
- 2 garlic cloves
- black pepper
- Balsamic vinegar
- Worcestershire sauce
- water

Directions:

1. Add all the ingredients to a pressure cooker in no particular order, and then add the spices and sauces to taste

2. Be sure to add enough water to cover the meat which will leave you with tender meat and some bone broth.
3. Set the cooker on the meat/stew option for at least two hours, depending on how well your mixture takes to it. Make sure the valve is set to close.
4. Do an instant release when the timer goes off.
5. Make sure you stir it often, so that there is not too much separation going on.
6. Add some salt and serve immediately.
7. It can also be stored in the fridge and reheated with some water.
8. Do not be worried when it turns to meat jelly in the fridge, as that means you did it right!

Pork Loin Carnivore Roast

Face it, nothing beats a nice roast. Perfect for any weather, but especially colder weather. A delicious carnivore-friendly recipe that will definitely be worth your while.

Time: 45 minutes

Serving Size: 9 servings

Prep Time: 10 minutes

Cook Time: 35 minutes

Nutritional Facts/Info:

Calories: 220

Carbs: 1 g

Fat: 7 g

Protein: 34 g

Ingredients:

- 3 lb pork loin roast
- 1 tsp onion powder
- 1 tsp dried oregano
- 1 tsp garlic powder
- 1 tsp ground cumin
- 1 tsp dried thyme
- 1 tsp coriander
- 1 tsp sea salt
- 1 tbsp oil
- 2 cloves garlic (minced)
- 2 cups chicken bone broth

Directions:

1. Mix the onion powder, oregano, garlic powder, cumin, thyme, coriander, and sea salt together in a small mixing bowl. Rub the mixed seasoning evenly into the pork loin roast.

2. Heat the oil in a pressure cooker on sauté then stir fry the minced garlic until you can smell it. Add the pork loin roast and brown all the sides.
3. Remove the roast and deglaze the pot with half of the chicken bone broth.
4. Add the remaining chicken bone broth then place the rack in the bottom of the pot. Place the pork loin roast on top of the rack.
5. Pressure cook on high for about 25 minutes. When it is done, do a quick pressure release. Remove the roast from the pot and allow it to sit for 10-15 minutes before slicing.

Carnivore Salmon with Garlic and Cilantro

Refreshing, convenient, and simply delicious!

Time: 25 minutes

Serving Size: 4 servings

Prep Time: 10 minutes

Cook Time: 15 minutes

Nutritional Facts/Info:

Calories: 210.2

Carbs: 0.4 g

Fat: 9.5 g

Protein: 29.0 g

Ingredients:

- 1 large salmon filet
- 1 lemon
- 4 garlic cloves (minced)
- ¼ cup fresh cilantro leaves (chopped)
- sea salt to taste
- black pepper to taste
- 1 tbsp butter

Directions:

1. Preheat the oven to 400°F. Place the salmon on a foil-lined baking sheet, skin side down. Do not grease the foil.
2. Squeeze the lemon over the salmon filet. Sprinkle the garlic and cilantro evenly over the top. Add the salt and pepper. Thinly slice the lemon and place the slices evenly over the top of the salmon filet.
3. Place the salmon with the foil in the preheated oven for about 7 minutes, depending on thickness.
4. Turn the oven up to broil and continue to cook for an additional 5-7 minutes, or until the top of the salmon filet is crispy.

5. Remove the salmon from the oven and slide a flat spatula in between the salmon and the skin. The skin should stick to the foil, easily separating the fish from its skin. Serve immediately.

Shrimp for the Grill

Light, yummy, quick and easy are the best ways to describe this dish. No fuss, and minimal messiness.

Time: 10 minutes

Serving Size: 4 servings

Prep Time: 10 minutes

Cook Time: 10 minutes

Nutritional Facts/Info:

Calories: 102

Carbs: 1 g

Fat: 3 g

Protein: 28 g

Ingredients:

For the seasoning:

- 1 tsp garlic powder
- 1 tsp sea salt
- 1 tsp Italian seasoning
- ½ tsp cayenne pepper

For the grill:

- 2 tbsp extra virgin olive oil
- 1 tbsp freshly-squeezed lemon juice
- 1 lb shrimp, peeled and deveined (jumbo)
- Canola oil for the grill

Directions:

1. Preheat a grill pan or an outdoor grill to high heat. To cook the shrimp in the oven, preheat the broiler. If broiling, line a baking sheet or pan with some foil and coat it with nonstick cooking spray.
2. In a medium-large mixing bowl, stir together the seasoning ingredients; garlic powder, salt, Italian seasoning, and cayenne. Add the olive oil and lemon juice and stir until it forms a paste.
3. Add the shrimp and toss it thoroughly to coat. If you are using smaller shrimp, stack them onto metal skewers or wooden skewers that have been soaked in water for at least 1 hour.

4. Brush the grill or grill pan with the Canola oil. Grill or broil the shrimp, just until they turn pink and opaque, for about 2 to 3 minutes on each side, turning once halfway through. Serve immediately for the best results.

Breakfast Sausage Patties

A delicious and hearty sausage recipe that is ideal for breakfast, lunch, or dinner. It has a low sodium count, and it can fit comfortably into your lunch box or fridge. You can even use the leftover juices from the skillet or pan to add some extra flavor to your next meal. Simply pour it into a container and pop it in the fridge. This sausage also pairs nicely with eggs and beef liver.

Time: 15 minutes

Serving Size: 4 servings

Prep Time: 5 minutes

Cook Time: 10 minutes

Nutritional Facts/Info:

Calories: 147.7

Carbs: 0.6 g

Fat: 11.1 g

Protein: 10.1 g

Ingredients:

- 8 oz fresh ground pork
- 2 tbsp chicken stock
- ½ tsp thyme (dried)
- ¼ tsp sage (dried)
- ½ tsp ground black pepper
- ½ tsp red pepper flakes

Directions:

1. Using your hands, carefully combine all ingredients in a mixing bowl.
2. Fold a sheet of waxed paper in half. Divide the sausage mixture into eight one-tablespoon portions and roll them into balls using your palms.
3. Place the balls on the waxed paper, fold over, and press down to compress the balls into patties.
4. Coat a non-stick skillet with cooking spray. Cook the patties over medium-high heat for 10 minutes, turning halfway. The sausage should cook until the internal temperature reaches 160°F.
5. Serve, and enjoy. Store any leftovers in the fridge.

Feta Chicken Patties

In the mood for a chicken burger? Try this delicious chicken and feta patty recipe. It is low-carb and extremely delicious. It can also be stored and reheated for another meal. It is ideal to take with you to a cookout. You can add it to your breakfast menu and top it with an egg or two. You can even use an indoor grill to prepare these delicious chicken patties.

Time: 20 minutes

Serving Size: 4 servings

Prep Time: 10 minutes

Cook Time: 10 minutes

Nutritional Facts/Info:

Calories: 285.6

Carbs: 3.3 g

Fat: 19.8 g

Protein: 26.8 g

Ingredients:
- 1 lb ground chicken
- 6 oz feta (crumbled)
- 1 tbsp ground oregano

- ¼ tsp salt
- ¼ tsp garlic powder

Directions:
1. Preheat the grill or broiler.
2. Mix all of the ingredients together in a large mixing bowl. Using your hands, roll the mixture into 4 equal-sized balls.
3. Press down on the balls with a decent amount of pressure to flatten them into formed patties. Repeat this method until you have 4 chicken patties.
4. Grill or broil the patties until their internal temperature reaches 165°F or cook them for about 7 to 8 minutes per side. Make sure they are cooked throughout.
5. Enjoy them as part of a meal, snack, or on the go.

Hickory Turkey Burgers

A scrumptious turkey burger goes a long way. Who said you need buns for the ideal turkey burger? Packed with protein and low-carb, this recipe will leave you wanting more. They are lighter than most burgers, so feel free to add them to your snack menu as well. They are easy to prepare and even easier to enjoy.

Time: 15 minutes

Serving Size: 4 servings

Prep Time: 5 minutes

Cook Time: 10 minutes

Nutritional Facts/Info:

Calories: 177.2

Carbs: 0.9 g

Fat: 8.6 g

Protein: 24.1 g

Ingredients:

- 1 lb ground turkey
- 1 dash salt
- 1 tsp liquid hickory flavored sauce (reduced sugar)
- 1 tsp garlic powder
- 1 tsp parsley
- 1 tsp paprika
- 1 tsp cumin powder
- 4 tbsp liquid egg substitute or 2 large beaten eggs

Directions:

1. Preheat the grill or fire up some coals to get started.
2. Using a medium or large mixing bowl, add all of the ingredients together and mix them together thoroughly.
3. Using your hands, roll the mixture into four equal-sized balls.
4. Press down on the balls to form equal-sized patties without causing them to break apart.
5. Store them in the fridge for a few minutes to set, or carefully place them on the grill.
6. Cook them for about 5 minutes on each side to ensure that they are cooked throughout. Use a spatula to ensure that they do not break apart as you grill them.
7. Serve and enjoy immediately or save them for later.

Chicken Pops

A truly fun and exciting new way to prepare chicken drumsticks, this is a simple recipe with a lot of flavor. If you are new in the kitchen, do not worry about pulling out the tendons. Creating these pops by moving the meat to the other end stops the bony end from drying out and burning before the meaty end is completely cooked.

Time: 56 minutes

Serving Size: 4 servings

Prep Time: 30 minutes

Cook Time: 26 minutes

Nutritional Facts/Info:

Calories: 187.8

Carbs: 5.6 g

Fat: 5.2 g

Protein: 29.8 g

Ingredients:
- 3 cloves garlic (minced)
- 1 shallot (minced)
- 1 tbsp low-sodium soy sauce
- 1 tsp mustard
- ¼ tsp ground black pepper
- ½ tsp turmeric
- ½ tsp paprika
- ¼ cup parsley leaves (finely chopped)
- 2 lemons (halved)
- 4 large chicken drumsticks, with the skin removed (about 4 ounces each)

Directions:

1. Mix together the first 8 ingredients along with the juice of half a lemon in a large mixing bowl.
2. Set aside about 3 tbsp of the mixture.
3. Preheat an outdoor grill to 400°F.
4. Place the chicken drumsticks on a cutting board. Using a sharpened chef's knife, cut the non-meat end around the bone turning the leg toward the knife. (Optional: Using small kitchen pliers, pull out the white tendons and discard them.)
5. Holding the bony end of the leg with one hand, use your other hand to gently push the meat up and toward the flesh end to form a "lollipop." Remove the remaining flesh from the bone by scraping it off with a knife.
6. Repeat the same technique with the rest of the drumsticks, placing each of them into the bowl with the marinade mixture as you finish prepping them.
7. Place the marinated drumsticks on the preheated grill, along with the remaining 3 lemon halves (flesh side facing down).
8. After 10 minutes, remove the lemons from the grill and turn the drumsticks. Grill the chicken for another 10 to 13 minutes, until they reach an internal temperature of 165°F.

9. When the lemons are cool enough to touch, squeeze them into the remaining sauce.
10. Pour the sauce over the pops and enjoy while they are still nice and warm.

Beef Chuck Roast

Here is a great way to cook a chuck roast that is fuss-free and extremely tender. Chuck can be a very flavorful roast and it does not have to be a tedious or difficult process. This delicious low-carb recipe is easy and convenient to follow, and the results are hearty and packed with nutrients. It is a great way to consume your protein.

Time: 1 hour 45 minutes

Serving Size: 8 servings

Prep Time: 5 minutes

Cook Time: 1 hour 40 minutes

Nutritional Facts/Info:

Calories: 212.1

Carbs: 0.7 g

Fat: 6.1 g

Protein: 36.3 g

Ingredients:

- 3 lb beef chuck (arm pot roast)
- 4 cloves garlic (peeled and halved)
- 1 tsp ground black pepper

Directions:

1. Preheat the oven to 400°F.
2. Secure the roast with cooking twine.
3. Make 8 slits of about ½ an inch each around the roast and insert half of a garlic clove into each cavity. Flavor with some fresh ground pepper and place it on a rack in a roasting pan.
4. Let it roast in the preheated oven for 20 minutes.
5. Reduce heat to 325°F and insert the meat thermometer into the roast.
6. Continue cooking for about 1 hour or until the roast is nice and tender. Do not overcook the roast, as it can become tough.
7. Remove it from the oven and loosely cover the roast with aluminum foil. Let it rest while covered for about 15 minutes before slicing or carving.
8. To serve, slice thinly against the grain, and use the pan drippings as gravy. If you wish to store

it in the fridge, make sure that it cools down completely before putting it away.

Lamb Chops for the Grill

This is another easy recipe ready for the kitchen or grill. Serve it warm for the best results. It is not necessary to marinate the chops ahead of time, but feel free to flavor them a few hours ahead of time and refrigerate. Take the chops out 30 minutes before grilling and have them reach room temperature before grilling.

Time: 26 minutes

Serving Size: 8 servings

Prep Time: 10 minutes

Cook Time: 6 minutes (+6-10 minutes to rest)

Nutritional Facts/Info:

Calories: 239

Carbs: 1 g

Fat: 16 g

Protein: 23 g

Ingredients:

- 8 lamb chops (about ¾ inch thickness)
- 3 tbsp extra virgin olive oil
- 1 tbsp fresh rosemary (finely chopped)
- 3 cloves garlic (minced)
- ½ tsp sea salt
- freshly ground black pepper to taste

Directions:

1. Preheat the grill or stove top grill pan to a medium-high heat.
2. Mix all the marinade ingredients together in a small mixing bowl. Spread this mixture evenly over all sides of the lamb chops.
3. Grill the lamb chops for 2 to 4 minutes on each side until they are tender (135°F for medium rare). Transfer the chops to a serving platter and let them rest for 6-10 minutes before serving.

Crispy Beef Liver

This recipe will leave you wanting more of these crispy, juicy beef livers. Ideal for sharing, but you might like them too much to share. Serve warm for the best results.

Time: 17 minutes

Serving Size: 5 servings

Prep Time: 10 minutes

Cook Time: 7 minutes

Nutritional Facts/Info:

Calories: 315

Carbs: 4 g

Fat: 25 g

Protein: 19 g

Ingredients:
- 1 lb beef liver (cut into thin slices)
- ½ cup olive oil
- 1 clove garlic (crushed)
- 1 tbsp fresh mint (chopped)
- 1 tsp sea salt
- ¼ tsp black pepper freshly ground

Directions:
1. Preheat a large grill pan over medium-high heat.
2. Rinse the liver under cold running water. Make sure to rinse out all of the blood. Pat it dry with a paper towel. Using a sharp knife, remove the rough veins, if there are any. Cut it crossways into thin slices.

3. In a small mixing bowl, combine the olive oil with the crushed garlic, mint, salt, and pepper. Mix until everything is well combined. Brush the liver slices with this mixture and grill for 5-7 minutes on each side.
4. Serve immediately for the best results.

Roast Beef Brisket

This is a roasted dish in all its glory. Share it with friends and family and enjoy the heartiness that it delivers. You will find this to be a dream meal for every carnivore.

Time: 4 hours 20 minutes

Serving Size: 10 servings

Prep Time: 20 minutes

Cook Time: 4 hours

Nutritional Facts/Info:

Calories: 369. 1

Carbs: 25.0 g

Fat: 10.1 g

Protein: 43.6 g

Ingredients:

- 4 lb beef brisket
- 2 tbsp olive oil
- 3 large onions
- 3 cloves garlic (minced)
- 3 stalks of celery
- 3 large carrots
- 1 small cabbage (chopped)
- 1 tsp bay leaf (crushed)
- 2-3 cups beef stock (homemade)
- 1 tsp mustard powder

Directions:

1. The day before you plan on serving the brisket, be sure to boil it in water to cover for 2 hours and refrigerate until the next day.
2. Preheat the oven to 300°F.
3. Add olive oil to a pan and brown the brisket on all sides. Once browned, set the brisket aside.
4. Add the garlic and onion to the pan and cook until brown.
5. Put the brisket in a baking dish, add all the ingredients, and cover.
6. Bake it for 4 hours, turning the brisket every hour (add water if necessary).
7. You can also make gravy from the leftover stock, and be sure to cut the meat against the grain before serving.

Broiled Parm Tilapia

This tilapia recipe is easy to make while you keep a watchful eye on the broiling time. Accessorize your weekly menu by trying out this low-carb tilapia recipe. This is an easy to prepare and quick carnivorous delight.

Time: 15 minutes

Serving Size: 4 servings

Prep Time: 5 minutes

Cook Time: 10 minutes

Nutritional Facts/Info:

Calories: 177.7

Carbs: 1.4 g

Fat: 8.3 g

Protein: 24.5 g

Ingredients:
- 1 lb tilapia fillets
- ¼ cup Parmesan cheese (shredded)
- 2 tbsp unsalted butter (softened)
- 1 tbsp plus ½ tsp reduced sugar mayonnaise
- 1 tbsp freshly squeezed lemon juice

- ⅛ tsp dried basil
- ⅛ tsp ground black pepper
- ⅛ tsp onion powder
- ⅛ tsp celery salt

Directions:

1. Preheat your oven's broiler. Grease a broiling pan or line with aluminum foil.
2. In a small mixing bowl, mix the Parmesan cheese, mayonnaise, butter, and lemon juice together.
3. Season the mixture with dried basil, onion powder, pepper, and celery salt. Mix well and set aside.
4. Place the fillets in a single layer on the prepared pan.
5. Broil the fillets a few inches away from the heat for 2-3 minutes.
6. Flip the fillets over and broil for an additional 2-3 minutes. Remove the fillets from the oven and cover them with the cheese mixture on the top.
7. Broil the fillets for another 2-3 minutes or until the topping is browned and the fish flakes easily with a fork.
8. Be careful not to overcook the fish as it could become dry or tough.

9. Let it cool down completely before storing it in the fridge. It is also best to let it breathe before covering it with any type of lid.

Marinated Flank Steak

Flank steak is affordable and flavorful, but it can be quite tough. This recipe will help you to cook the juiciest, tastiest, and most tender flank steak you have ever tasted. Marinade it before cooking and cut your cooked steak against the grain to maintain its tender qualities.

Time: 30 minutes

Serving Size: 4 servings

Prep Time: 10 minutes

Cook Time: 20 minutes

Nutritional Facts/Info:

Calories: 215

Carbs: 2.9 g

Fat: 11.8 g

Protein: 23.5 g

Ingredients:

- ½ cup salsa
- 1 clove garlic (minced)
- 1 tbsp olive oil
- 1 lime
- 1 lb flank steak

Directions:

1. Put the salsa, garlic, olive oil, and lime juice in a zip top bag. Shake the ingredients in the bag to mix everything thoroughly.
2. Add the flank steak to the mixture in the bag. Re-seal the bag after letting out as much air as possible. Let the steak marinade in the fridge for at least 4 hours.
3. When it is time to cook the steak, remove it from the zip top bag, and discard the marinade.
4. Grill or broil the flank steak to your preference (medium, rare, well-done, etc.); however, keep in mind that flank steak can become extremely tough if it is overcooked.
5. Let it rest for about 10 minutes, and then slice the meat against the grain into thin slices. Serve immediately.

Carnivore Beef Broth

Consuming bone broth is one of the best ways to nourish your body while following the carnivore diet. This recipe is quick and easy to follow right in your own kitchen. Remember to use grass-fed beef marrow bones for the best results.

Time: 24 hours 10 minutes

Serving Size: 16 servings

Prep Time: 10 minutes

Cook Time: 24 hours

Nutritional Facts/Info:

Calories: 69.2

Carbs: 0.8 g

Fat: 4.0 g

Protein: 6.4 g

Ingredients:
- 2 lb grass-fed marrow bones
- 1 gallon filtered water
- 2 tbsp organic apple cider vinegar
- 1 tsp sea salt (to taste)
- 12 garlic cloves

Directions:
1. Brown the marrow bones in a greased pan to add some flavor.
2. Add all the ingredients into a crock pot. Cook it on high until the broth starts to boil, then switch it to low and cook for an additional 10-24 hours. Remember, longer is always better when it comes to broth.
3. Let the broth cool, and then transfer it to glass jars or any containers of your choice. Store it in the fridge for a few days or freeze it if you would like to keep it longer.

Freezer/Reheating Friendly

Carnivore Steak Nuggets

Quick and delicious, this dish is fun to eat and easy to store. Make several batches of these steak nuggets and store them raw, in the freezer. They can be stored frozen for about 6 months. To cook, fry from frozen.

Time: 40 minutes

Serving Size: 4 servings

Prep Time: 35 minutes

Cook Time: 5 minutes

Nutritional Facts/Info:

Calories: 350

Carbs: 1 g

Fat: 200 g

Protein: 40 g

Ingredients:

- 1 lb venison or beef steak cut into chunks
- 1 large egg
- Lard or palm oil

Breading

- ½ cup grated Parmesan cheese
- ½ cup pork panko
- ½ tsp homemade seasoned salt

Dip (optional)

- ¼ cup mayonnaise
- ¼ cup sour cream (organic, cultured)
- 1+ tsp chipotle paste to taste
- ½ tsp homemade ranch dressing and dip mix
- ¼ medium lime (juiced)

Directions:

1. For the dip: Combine all of the ingredients and mix it thoroughly. 1 tsp of the chipotle paste produces a medium-spice variety; use more or less according to taste. Refrigerate 30 minutes before serving and remember that it can be kept refrigerated for up to 1 week.
2. Combine the pork panko, Parmesan cheese and seasoned salt and set aside.
3. Beat 1 egg and place the beaten egg in a mixing bowl and the breading mix in another.
4. Dip the cut pieces of steak in the egg, and follow with the breading. Place it on a wax paper lined sheet pan or plate.
5. Freeze the breaded raw steak bites for 30 minutes before frying. This way, the breading will not pull away from the meat while frying.
6. Heat the lard or oil to roughly 325°F. Fry the steak nuggets (from frozen) until browned, for about 2-3 minutes.
7. Transfer to a paper towel lined dish, flavor with a sprinkle of salt, and serve it with or without the dip.

Freezer Breakfast Sandwiches

There are few things as convenient and easy to make as these breakfast sandwiches. As these are sandwiches, keto-friendly bread is a great substitute, or you can just skip the bread part entirely.

Time: 20 minutes

Serving Size: 8 servings

Prep Time: 5 minutes

Cook Time: 15 minutes

Nutritional Facts/Info:

Calories: 304.8

Carbs: 10 g

Fat: 14. 2 g

Protein: 24.6 g

Ingredients:
- 8 large eggs
- 1 tsp sea salt
- 1 tsp ground black pepper
- 8 keto-friendly buns
- 8 x 1 oz slices Swiss cheese
- 3 oz buffalo chicken

- 3 oz roast beef

Directions:
1. Preheat the oven to 350°F.
2. Spray a muffin tin with cooking spray and crack an egg into each of 8 cups.
3. Season with sea salt and ground black pepper.
4. Bake for 10-15 minutes depending on your preference.
5. In the meantime, prepare 8 sandwich-size freezer bags, placing a keto-friendly bun (cut open) on each piece.
6. Add ¾ oz meat to each sandwich; half chicken and half beef.
7. Add a slice of Swiss cheese to each sandwich.
8. When the eggs are done, remove them from the oven and let them cool for 2-4 minutes.
9. Scoop one egg onto each sandwich and prepare it for the freezer.
10. When you are ready to eat them, remove them from the freezer and heat it in the microwave for a few minutes.

Beefy Taco Pie

This taco pie can easily be frozen for future use. Bake it first and then freeze it for the best results. To prepare it for freezing, cut it into slices and cover with foil.

Time: 45 minutes

Serving Size: 8 servings

Prep Time: 10 minutes

Cook Time: 35 minutes

Nutritional Facts/Info:

Calories: 268

Carbs: 2 g

Fat: 20 g

Protein: 19 g

Ingredients:

- 1 lb ground beef (grass-fed)
- 1 packet taco seasoning (free of MSG, starches, and additives)
- 3 green onions (thinly sliced)
- ¼ cup salsa

- 1 cup Mexican blend cheese (shredded, quantity divided)
- 4 large eggs
- 2/3 cup heavy cream, preferably grass-fed
- ½ teaspoon sea salt

Directions:

1. Preheat the oven to 350°F. Prepare a round deep dish or pie dish by greasing it with butter.
2. Heat a large skillet over medium-high heat. Be sure the beef is not low in fat to yield the best cooking results. When the skillet is hot, add the ground beef, breaking it into small pieces with a spatula. Stir it occasionally until it is browned.
3. Drain the beef and stir in the taco seasoning. Set it aside.
4. In a medium-sized mixing bowl, stir together the eggs and the heavy cream. Stir in the salsa, green onions, ¾ cup of the cheese, and the salt.
5. Stir the prepared taco meat into the egg mixture. Pour the entire mixture into the prepared pie pan. Sprinkle some of the remaining cheese on top.
6. Bake the pie in the preheated oven for 35-45 minutes or until the top is brown and the pie is completely set. Allow it to cool for 5 minutes before serving. Serve it with some other taco toppings or enjoy it as it is.

Organ Meat Pie

Organ meats are some of the more affordable meats and are also some of the most nutritious meats as well. This nourishing recipe combination of ground beef, heart, and liver is baked into a meat pie. This is an easy, delicious, and satisfying meal.

Time: 20 minutes

Serving Size: 4 servings

Prep Time: 5 minutes

Cook Time: 15 minutes

Nutritional Facts/Info:

Calories: 412

Carbs: 2 g

Fat: 28 g

Protein: 35 g

Ingredients:

- ½ lb ground beef
- ½ lb ground beef heart
- ½ lb ground beef liver
- beef tallow, butter, or ghee
- 3 eggs

- sea salt

Directions:
1. Preheat the oven to 350°F.
2. Combine all of the ingredients in a large mixing bowl. Add sea salt to taste.
3. Distribute the mixture evenly into a lightly greased 9-inch pie plate.
4. Bake the dish for about 15-20 minutes, until the egg is set.
5. Remove it from the oven, and let it cool for 5 minutes. Serve warm and/or freeze in a freezer-friendly container for up to 3 months.

Herb Roasted Bone Marrow

Bone marrow is a most beneficial addition to the carnivore diet. It is filled with dense nutrients that can optimize your health and tastes amazing at the same time. This recipe is ideal for those days when you need a boost. Bone marrow can also be kept frozen for quite some time.

Time: 20 minutes

Serving Size: 1 serving

Prep Time: 5 minutes

Cook Time: 15 minutes

Nutritional Facts/Info:

Calories: 110

Carbs: 1 g

Fat: 12 g

Protein: 5 g

Ingredients:

- Marrow bones from grass-fed/pasture-raised beef
- Fresh rosemary
- Fresh thyme
- Unrefined salt
- Ground black pepper

Directions:

1. If you have purchased frozen bones, make sure to thaw them completely in the fridge before cooking. Preheat the oven to 400°F degrees. Place the bones in a baking dish or cast iron pan.
2. Using a sharp knife, chop equal parts of fresh rosemary and thyme. You can also use ½ tsp of chopped herbs for every 4 marrow bones.

Sprinkle the herbs over the marrow bones and make sure each one is covered.
3. Roast the bones for about 15 minutes, or until they are no longer pink inside.
4. Season the bones with salt and pepper and serve hot. Use a small spoon to scoop out the marrow. You can also keep the residue liquid in the pan in an airtight container in the fridge to add to your other meals for added flavor.

Chicken Gizzards and Broth

A lot of people give gizzards a hard time when, in fact, they are tender and delicious. This recipe is designed to highlight the many flavors and nutrients that gizzards can provide. You can also save this meal in the freezer and heat it later.

Time: 35 minutes

Serving Size: 4 servings

Prep Time: 5 minutes

Cook Time: 35 minutes

Nutritional Facts/Info:

Calories: 79

Carbs: 3 g

Fat: 8 g

Protein: 1 g

Ingredients:

- 1 lb chicken gizzards (cut into quarters)
- 2 tbsp ghee
- 1 medium onion (chopped)
- 2 cloves garlic (chopped finely)
- 1 tsp sea salt
- ¼ tsp ground black pepper
- 4 cups water

Directions:

1. Using the sauté setting on your pressure cooker, sauté the onions, garlic, and gizzards.
2. Cook the mixture until the onions are translucent and gizzards no longer look raw, then add in your water. Make sure to stir it occasionally.
3. Put the lid on the cooker and cook the dish at high pressure for 25 minutes.
4. Allow it to naturally depressurize before opening. Garnish the dish with chives and/or chive blossoms (optional).

Carnivore Freezer Pizza

In the mood for pizza? This pizza recipe is ideal for freezing and reheating when you feel like it. It is a low-carb, high-protein and fat alternative for standard Italian pizza and the best way to curb cravings. Going carnivore does not have to be a bland experience, especially not when you have recipes like this at hand. Prepare 3 pizzas at a time, for example, and keep them in the freezer. In this way, you can save time and effort.

Time: 30 minutes

Serving Size: 8 servings

Prep Time: 15 minutes

Cook Time: 15 minutes

Nutritional Facts/Info:

Calories: 228.8

Carbs: 1.2 g

Fat: 18.6 g

Protein: 15.6 g

Ingredients:
- 2 tbsp ranch dressing (reduced sugar)
- 12 oz ground beef (not lean)

- 1 serving pepperoni (13 pieces)
- 2 cups mozzarella cheese
- 2 cups diced bacon
- 1 low-carb or keto tortilla (large)

Directions:

1. Preheat the oven to 400°F.
2. Place a tortilla on a greased baking sheet. Add the ranch dressing and spread it evenly all over the tortilla surface.
3. Continue to add the cheese, beef, pepperoni, and diced bacon. Make sure all of the ingredients are spaced out evenly so that they cover the entire pizza surface.
4. Place the pizza in the oven and bake it for 15 minutes until the cheese is melted and the toppings are a light golden brown. Serve warm or let it cool down for about an hour and place it in the freezer.
5. To reheat, take it out of the freezer and put it in the oven at 400°F for 5-10 minutes.

Yummy Meatloaf

A protein-rich recipe that can be enjoyed now or frozen and saved for a later time. It is easy to store and even easier to prepare. Be sure not to overcook it to avoid dryness, but do give it time to set for the best result. This is also a great recipe for those who like to pack leftovers for lunch or dinner. Enjoy it with friends or family.

Time: 1 hour 10 minutes

Serving Size: 12 servings

Prep Time: 10 minutes

Cook Time: 1 hour

Nutritional Facts/Info:

Calories: 134. 5

Carbs: 1.1 g

Fat: 5.0 g

Protein: 20.0 g

Ingredients:
- 2.2 lb ground beef
- 1 onion (finely chopped)
- 2 large eggs (beaten)
- 4 tbsp plain full-fat yoghurt
- 2 hard-boiled eggs (sliced)
- sea salt and ground black pepper to taste
- 1 tsp crushed garlic

Directions:
1. Preheat the oven to 350°F.
2. Mix together the chopped onion, beaten eggs, yogurt, and season with the salt, pepper, and garlic. Add the ground beef into the mixture and stir again.
3. Lightly grease a bread tin with non-stick spray. Do not use oil or butter, as this could cause the dish to become too oily.
4. Add the mixture and the sliced boiled eggs into the bread tin and put it into the oven.
5. Cook the meatloaf for one hour. Let the loaf stand for 10 minutes before slicing so that it can set.
6. Serve hot or store it in the freezer for another day.

Cocoa Crusted Pork Tenderloin

This dish is inspired by Costa Rican spices. It seems exotic, but you can use spices and ingredients you already have on hand like coffee, cocoa, and cinnamon. It is a sweet approach to a lovely pork tenderloin. It can also be frozen and reheated in the microwave or oven for later consumption. You will not be able to get enough of this one. It is also protein rich which is something that should be considered in the carnivore diet.

Time: 18-20 minutes

Serving Size: 4 servings

Prep Time: 3-5 minutes

Cook Time: 15 minutes

Nutritional Facts/Info:

Calories: 264.0

Carbs: 1.2 g

Fat: 13.1 g

Protein: 33.7 g

Ingredients:

- 1 tbsp cocoa powder (unsweetened)
- 1 tsp instant coffee
- ½ tsp cinnamon powder
- ½ tsp chili powder
- 1 tbsp butter
- 1 lb pork tenderloin (trimmed)

Directions:

1. Preheat the oven to 400°F degrees.
2. Combine all of the spices in a mixing bowl. Prepare the pork tenderloin by removing the

thin silver tendon that may be running down the centre of the loin.
3. Rub the tenderloin with butter. Season the loin with all of the spice mixture. Heat a cast iron or heavy-bottomed pan to high heat. Spray with non-stick cooking spray.
4. Place the tenderloin in the pan and sear on both sides. Transfer the pan to the oven and roast for 15 minutes or until the internal temperature reaches 145°F.
5. Remove the pan from the oven and place the meat on a cutting board and allow it to rest for 5 minutes before slicing.
6. Enjoy at any time or freeze for later consumption.

Easy Roast Beef

Versatile, easy, and carnivore-friendly, this recipe can be your go-to meal prep favorite. Prepare this roast on a Sunday and enjoy it throughout the week. You can add some salt if you prefer a saltier roast and some garlic for added flavor. However, it is equally enjoyable with black pepper only. Freeze or refrigerate it and reheat it in the microwave or oven for a quick meal.

Time: 1 hour 20 minutes

Serving Size: 12 servings

Prep Time: 10 minutes

Cook Time: 1 hour 10 minutes

Nutritional Facts/Info:

Calories: 191.2

Carbs: 0.1 g

Fat: 7.6 g

Protein: 28.7 g

Ingredients:
- 2 ½ lb top round beef roast
- 1 tsp cracked black pepper

Directions:
1. Preheat the oven to 400° F.
2. Remove the meat from the refrigerator and allow it to rest at room temperature for about 20 minutes.
3. Pat the meat dry with paper towels to remove any moisture. Season with black pepper and then rub the pepper over the meat.
4. Place a cast-iron skillet or heavy ovenproof sauté pan over moderate heat. Do not add cooking spray or any oil to the pan, as there is no grease required at moderate heat. Sear the

meat on all sides, then move the pan to the oven.
5. Reduce the oven temperature to 350°F and roast it until the internal temperature reaches 125°F; this will take about 50 minutes. Remove the meat from the oven, cover with foil, and let it rest for 10 minutes before carving into thin slices.
6. Store for later consumption or enjoy throughout the day.

Easy Seafood Stock

It is easy to find healthy chicken and beef stocks in stores. On the other hand, a good seafood stock is not that easy to find. This recipe makes a delicious seafood stock that can be frozen. It is a great source of nutrients and flavor and can liven up any meal.

Time: 35 minutes

Serving Size: 8 servings

Prep Time: 10 minutes

Cook Time: 25 minutes

Nutritional Facts/Info:

Calories: 18.7

Carbs: 3.2 g

Fat: 0.6 g

Protein: 0.5 g

Ingredients:

- 4 oz shrimp shells (from about 15-20 shrimp)
- 1 tsp soybean oil
- ¾ cup onion (chopped)
- 1 leek, white and pale green part only (thinly sliced)
- 1 stalk celery (chopped)
- 6 peppercorns
- 4-½ cups cold water

Directions:

1. Heat a stock pot or large saucepan over moderate heat.
2. Add the oil to the hot pan, then add the shrimp shells to the hot oil.
3. Sauté until the shells become bright pink or reddish in color. Add the vegetables and stir to combine. Reduce the heat to low and let it sweat for 3 minutes.
4. Add the seasonings and water and turn the heat up to high. Bring the stock to a boil, and then lower the heat and simmer for 20-25 minutes.

5. Set it aside and let it cool slightly. Then, strain the stock through a fine-mesh strainer.
6. Add to a container of your preference and store it in the fridge or freezer.

Slow Cooker Carnivore Beef Stew

This collagen-packed, extra meaty carnivore beef stew is slow cooked in a crockpot. It is filled with flavor from low-carb vegetables and herbs. This stew is deeply nourishing and suitable for any day of the week, freezer-friendly, and takes minimal effort to prepare.

Time: 8 hours 20 minutes

Serving Size: 6 servings

Prep Time: 20 minutes

Cook Time: 8 hours

Nutritional Facts/Info:

Calories: 509

Carbs: 6 g

Fat: 28 g

Protein: 38 g

Ingredients:

- 2 lb beef marrow bones
- 2 lb chuck roast cubed
- 2 tbsp beef tallow
- 6 cups bone broth
- 8 oz mushrooms (quartered)
- 1 large onion chopped
- 4 cloves garlic minced
- 2 tsp dried thyme
- 2 tsp salt
- 1 tsp ground black pepper

Directions:

1. Start the slow cooker on a low setting and place the marrow bones in the centre.
2. Cube the roast and heat the tallow in a large skillet over high heat. Arrange the meat in a single layer and sear on all sides. Once all the meat is cooked, add it to the pot.
3. Rinse and chop all of the vegetables, gather the herbs, and place everything in the pot on top of the meat.
4. Pour the broth over the ingredients and season with salt and pepper.
5. Cover with the lid and cook on low for 6-8 hours.
6. Set it aside and let it cool down before freezing it in freezer-friendly containers. Freeze it in

separate containers and heat it up in the oven or microwave when you are ready to enjoy.

Simple Liver and Onions

This tasty, nutrient-dense and easy liver recipe can be frozen and stored easily. The carnivore diet encourages eating a lot of liver due to its high fat and protein content. It is also very delicious and can be extremely filling. Reheat it in the microwave or oven and enjoy it whenever you feel the urge. It is a great source of nutrients and utterly delicious.

Time: 35 minutes

Serving Size: 6 servings

Prep Time: 15 minutes

Cook Time: 20 minutes

Nutritional Facts/Info:

Calories: 186. 4

Carbs: 7.7 g

Fat: 9.7 g

Protein: 14.7 g

Ingredients:

- 1 lb calf liver
- 1 medium onion (chopped)
- 1 tbsp extra virgin olive oil
- ¼ cup flour (optional)
- 1 tsp black pepper
- ¼ tsp garlic powder
- 1-2 cups of water

Directions:

1. Heat the oil in a skillet. Flour the pieces of liver (optional) and place in the skillet.
2. Brown the liver on both sides and remove it from the pan.
3. Add the onions and garlic powder and sauté until the onions are clear. Add some flour, one tablespoon at a time, until the oil is absorbed, and the flour is lightly browned.
4. Add the water to flour and onion mixture until it reaches a gravy consistency according to your preference.
5. Let it simmer for about 5 minutes and then return the liver to the pan. Cover with a lid and let it simmer for another 10-15 minutes.
6. Note that you do not have to add flour, as the recipe tastes great without it. You can also substitute the flour with some finely grated Parmesan cheese. If you do choose flour, please note that this dish should not be enjoyed often

if you choose to follow the carnivore diet religiously, as it is higher in carbohydrates than recommended.

Freezer-Friendly Italian Meatballs

This recipe makes irresistible Italian meatballs that are perfectly delicious and convenient in the best ways possible. Enjoy them any time of the day as a snack or even a meal. Take them with you anywhere and reheat them in a microwave for the best results.

Time: 1 hour

Serving Size: 6 servings

Prep Time: 20 minutes

Cook Time: 40 minutes

Nutritional Facts/Info:

Calories: 404

Carbs: 4 g

Fat: 28 g

Protein: 28 g

Ingredients:

- ½ cup Parmesan cheese (finely grated)
- ½ cup full fat milk
- 1 lb ground beef
- 1 lb ground pork sausage
- 1 egg
- 2 tsp dried parsley
- 1 tsp dried Italian seasoning blend
- ½ tsp salt
- ¼ tsp pepper

Directions:

1. Line a large cookie sheet with foil and set aside.
2. Add the milk to the Parmesan cheese and let it soak for 5 minutes.
3. In a large mixing bowl add both of the meats along with the seasonings and the egg.
4. Add the soaked Parmesan cheese to the meats.
5. Using your hands gently mix everything together until it is well combined. Be careful not to overwork.
6. Using an ice cream scoop or similar type of spoon, scoop the meat mixture into your hands and gently roll it into balls.
7. Place the balls on the foil-lined cookie sheet and repeat until all of the meat mixture is used.
8. Place the cookie sheet in the oven and turn on the broiler.

9. Broil for about 8 minutes until they are lightly browned and crispy and then carefully flip the meatballs and broil for an additional 4 minutes.
10. Reduce the oven's heat to 400°F and let the meatballs continue to cook for an additional 10 minutes or until they are cooked through.
11. Remove them from the oven and let them cool completely.
12. Transfer the cooked meatballs to a clean parchment paper-lined cookie sheet.
13. Place them in the freezer for about 2 hours or until they are set and firm.
14. Transfer meatballs to a bag or container and return them to the freezer for up to 4 months.
15. To reheat, simply place them in the microwave or oven for a few minutes.

Bacon Meatloaf Muffins

This is another easy, convenient, and tasty carnivore meal that can be frozen without hesitation and saved for a rainy day. It is perfect for the whole family and packed with the nutrients that your body requires. Ideal for an on-the-go breakfast, lunch, or dinner and even a great fit for your lunchbox.

Time: 35 minutes

Serving Size: 8 servings

Prep Time: 15 minutes

Cook Time: 20 minutes

Nutritional Facts/Info:

Calories: 190.8

Carbs: 2 g

Fat: 15.8 g

Protein: 10.2 g

Ingredients:
- 1 lb ground beef
- 3 cloves garlic (minced)
- ¼ onion (minced)
- 2 tbsp Worcestershire sauce
- 1 tbsp Italian seasoning
- 2 slices bacon (cut into 8 pieces)

Sauce:
- ¼ cup reduced sugar tomato sauce
- 1 tbsp raw honey
- ½ tbsp mustard
- 2 slices bacon, cut into 8 pieces

Directions:
1. Preheat the oven to 350°F.

2. Mix together all of the filling ingredients. Place the filling into 8 cups of a muffin pan and top with sauce and then a piece of bacon.
3. Bake for 15 minutes and then broil for an additional 2-3 minutes until the bacon is crispy.
4. Pour some of the fat into a container and store it for cooking later.
5. Let everything cool down before removing from the pan. Store them separately for easier reheating in freezer-friendly containers or bags.
6. Simply pop them in the microwave for 1-2 minutes to reheat and enjoy.
7. Makes eight muffin-sized servings.

Slow Cooker Beef Strips

A quick and easy slow-cooker recipe ideal for freezing and reheating, these hearty beef strips are ideal for a snack, meal, or quick meal. Make sure you let them cool down entirely before you put them in the freezer to prevent the juices from separating during the freezing process. Reheat them in the microwave for a few minutes and enjoy. They are easy to store and grab as you go.

Time: 3 hours 5 minutes

Serving Size: 4 servings

Prep Time: 5 minutes

Cook Time: 3 hours

Nutritional Facts/Info:

Calories: 191.1

Carbs: 4 g

Fat: 4.5 g

Protein: 29.9 g

Ingredients:
- 1 lb top or bottom round steak (thinly sliced)
- 1 large onion (chopped)
- 4 tbsp soy sauce
- 1 tbsp garlic powder
- ¼ cup water
- 1 beef bouillon cube

Directions:
1. Cut the round steaks in 1-inch strips and do not remove the excess fat.
2. Place the strips in the crock pot. Add the onion, garlic powder, bouillon cube, and soy sauce on top of the strips in the crock pot. Pour the water over the meat mixture. Cook on high for 2.5-3 hours or low for 6 hours.

Fish Nuggets

Here is a yummy fish recipe that is convenient, easy, and freezer-friendly. Use pork rinds for some added flavor and let the nuggets cool down entirely before storing them in the freezer. You can simply reheat them in the microwave for a few minutes and enjoy them at home, work, or school. These little nuggets should not be underestimated, as they are delicious and nutritious.

Time: 20 minutes

Serving Size: 3 servings

Prep Time: 15 minutes

Cook Time: 5 minutes

Nutritional Facts/Info:

Calories: 432.7

Carbs: 0.9 g

Fat: 24.3 g

Protein: 50.6 g

Ingredients:
- ½ cup of finely ground pork rinds
- ½ cup Parmesan cheese (grated)
- 1 tsp sea salt and black pepper

- ½ tsp cayenne pepper
- ½ tsp garlic powder
- 1 egg
- 1 tbsp heavy cream
- 3 frozen vacuum-sealed Tilapia fillets
- 3 tbsp extra virgin olive oil

Directions:

1. Thaw the fish by letting the still vacuum-sealed fillets sit in a bowl of hot water for a few minutes.
2. Use a food processor to finely ground the pork rinds into a powder, so that it can stick to the fish easily.
3. In a large mixing bowl, mix the pork rind powder with the Parmesan and all of the spices. Make sure to mix everything together well for even distribution.
4. In a second mixing bowl, whisk together the egg and heavy cream.
5. Cut the thawed fish into 1-inch nuggets. The smaller the nuggets, the faster they will cook, and the less the chance of the "breading" being burned.
6. Heat a skillet to medium-high heat, and then add enough oil to coat the entire surface to a depth of about ¼ inch.

7. Coat the fish pieces in the egg mixture on all sides, and then coat them in the pork rind/cheese mixture and add them to the oil.
8. Fry the nuggets until they are golden brown, for about 2-3 minutes, flipping them halfway through to ensure consistency.
9. Let them cool down before popping them in the freezer and place them in the microwave to reheat them.

Chili Cheese Dog Casserole

Here is something to spice up your pallet a little bit. This casserole is suited for those who like to live life on the spicier side. You can store portions of this casserole separately and reheat them in the oven or microwave before lunch or dinner. With all this flavor, you will not feel as if you are missing out on anything. It is also ideal for colder months because it warms you up from the inside.

Time: 50 minutes

Serving Size: 10 servings

Prep Time: 30 minutes

Cook Time: 20 minutes

Nutritional Facts/Info:

Calories: 339.5

Carbs: 3 g

Fat: 25.9 g

Protein: 24.5 g

Ingredients:

- 2 tsp chili powder
- 1 tsp cumin powder
- ½ tsp sea salt
- ½ cup onions (chopped)
- 1 cup cheddar cheese (finely shredded)
- 2 lb ground beef chuck
- 9 uncured beef hot dogs
- 1 cup natural tomato sauce
- 2 tbsp tomato paste (sugar free)
- 2 tbsp Worcestershire sauce

Directions:

1. Preheat the oven to 400°F.
2. Brown the beef and add some salt while cooking. Mix all of the spices in a small bowl along with the sauce and tomato paste.
3. Once the beef is cooked, drain any excess moisture and set aside.

4. Add the hot dogs to the pan and brown. Let them cool down and then cut them in half, carrying on slicing them into ½-inch pieces.
5. In a large mixing bowl, combine the beef, hot dogs, onions, tomato, and spices and spread into a 9"x13" casserole dish. Top it with cheese and cook it for 20 minutes. If the mixture seems too dry, you can add some water.
6. Let it cool down completely before storing or freezing.

Snacks

Liver and Bacon Cups

Having these on hand as a snack is definitely a must if you intend on taking the carnivore diet seriously. This nutritious muffin-type snack will curb your hunger and cravings. Store them in the fridge for up to three days. They will also fit into a small lunchbox quite easily.

Time: 40 minutes

Serving Size: 12 servings

Prep Time: 10 minutes

Cook Time: 30 minutes

Nutritional Facts/Info:

Calories: 137

Carbs: 1 g

Fat: 7 g

Protein: 17 g

Ingredients:

- 12 oz grass fed ground beef
- 12 oz beef liver
- 12 oz bacon
- ¼ cup bone broth
- 1 tsp oregano
- 1 tsp thyme
- 1 tsp rosemary
- 1 tsp salt

Directions:

1. Preheat the oven to 350°F.
2. Using a pan or skillet, cook the bacon until it is tender, saving some bacon grease for later use.
3. Blend the cooked bacon and liver together to a semi-even texture.
4. Transfer to a large mixing bowl and add in the ground beef.

5. Flavor the mixture with the bone broth and herbs.
6. Add the mixture into a muffin pan and bake it for roughly 30 minutes.
7. Serve and enjoy or store for later.

Meaty French Fries

You do not have to worry about carbohydrates with this recipe for meaty French fries, because there are none. They can be enjoyed as a snack or even a side dish for a carnivore meal. A guilt-free approach to substituting French fries.

Time: 40 minutes

Serving Size: 1 serving

Prep Time: 10-15 minutes

Cook Time: 25-30 minutes

Nutritional Facts/Info:

Calories: 248

Carbs: 0 g

Fat: 10 g

Protein: 38 g

Ingredients:

- 4 oz cooked poultry (feel free to use light and dark meat chicken)
- ⅛ cup pork rinds
- 1 whole egg
- ¼ tsp salt
- ¼ tsp baking powder

Directions:

1. Preheat the oven to 350ºF.
2. Line a baking dish with parchment paper.
3. Blend all of the ingredients together until the mixture is evenly mixed.
4. Stuff the mixture into a plastic bag and cut a small hole in a corner so that you can squeeze the fries onto the parchment paper.
5. Squeeze out your preferred size of fries and then compress and shape them. Once you are happy with the shape, bake them in the oven for 15-20 minutes.
6. Afterwards, broil them on high for 2-3 minutes until they are golden and crispy on top, just like potato fries.
7. One serving should amount to 12-15 thick cut fries. They taste their best when they are warm.

Chicken Chips

Crispy, crackling, refreshing and packed with protein and fat, this is the ideal snack for those carnivores who truly miss the crunchiness of potato chips. They are extremely easy to store or take with you anywhere you go. Pack them in an airtight container and you are off! Another easy-to-follow carnivore delight.

Time: 25 minutes

Serving Size: 1 serving

Prep Time: 5 minutes

Cook Time: 20 minutes

Nutritional Facts/Info:

Calories: 154

Carbs: 0 g

Fat: 3.9 g

Protein: 6.9 g

Ingredients:

- chicken skin (from one whole chicken)
- 1 tsp sea salt
- 1 tsp cayenne pepper seasoning

Directions:

1. Take all the skin off of the whole chicken, rinse the skin with water only, and gently pat it dry.
2. Once the skin is dry, cut it into chip shapes like squares, triangles, or ovals.
3. Place the cut skin on a sheet of parchment paper and season it with the sea salt and the cayenne pepper. If cayenne pepper is not desired, then use only the salt.
4. Place another piece of parchment paper on top of the seasoned skin and place a baking pan on top to keep them flat while they are baking.
5. Bake at 400°F for 10 minutes at first and then turn them over to bake for another 8-10 minutes until they are nice and crispy.
6. Serve and enjoy.

Party Paté

This is a delicious liver paté containing bison and pork belly. It does sound a little bit fancy, but do not be fooled. It is extremely easy to prepare and suitable for all cooking levels. If you are not the paté type, you can even incorporate it into another meal to amplify the taste and boost the nutrition. Liver paté is a great source of nutrients especially for carnivores. It is also a convenient snack.

Time: 20 minutes

Serving Size: 4 servings

Prep Time: 5 minutes

Cook Time: 10-20 minutes

Nutritional Facts/Info:

Calories: 173

Carbs: 0 g

Fat: 15.8 g

Protein: 7.2 g

Ingredients:
- 3 oz beef liver
- 3 oz pork belly
- 1 tsp ghee
- 1 tsp sea salt (to taste)

Directions:
1. Cook the pork belly and remove from the pan. Sauté the liver in the pork belly fat in a skillet or pan until the outside is properly cooked, but the inside is still somewhat pinkish.

2. Add the pork belly, liver, ghee, and sea salt (to taste) to a blender or food processor. Blend everything until it has a smooth consistency.
3. You can save some of the fat left in the skillet or pan to cook with later.
4. Store the paté in the fridge and thin it out with some bone broth when you are ready to use it. It goes great with eggs too.

Egg Loaf Muffins

These yummy egg loaf muffins are the perfect low-carb/keto/carnivore-friendly snack. The recipe makes three medium-sized muffins or 6 mini muffins. It all depends on the size of the muffin pan that you choose. These muffins are easy to make and pack some serious flavor. Add them to your lunchbox and take them with you. You never know when they might come in handy.

Time: 20 minutes

Serving Size: 3 medium-sized muffins or 6 mini muffins (2 servings)

Prep Time: 10 minutes

Cook Time: 10 minutes

Nutritional Facts/Info:

Calories: 421

Carbs: 1 g

Fat: 17 g

Protein: 8 g

Ingredients:

- 2 oz cream cheese
- 2 eggs
- 2-½ tsp grass-fed ghee
- 1 dash of unsweetened almond milk
- ½ tsp baking powder
- ½ tsp cinnamon
- ½ tsp stevia
- sea salt to taste

Directions:

1. Preheat the oven to 375°F and prepare a muffin pan with non-stick spray.
2. Using a blender, combine all the ingredients and blend until evenly smooth.
3. Add a bit of almond milk to liquify the batter. Do not add too much.
4. If you do not have a blender, you can mix ingredients together with a tablespoon; just start

by mixing the cream cheese with the almond milk first in order to soften it and remove any lumps, and then add the rest of the ingredients and mix well.
5. Continue to pour the mixture into the muffin pan and put it in the oven for 8-10 minutes or until the muffins are puffed.
6. Serve and enjoy.

Angel Food Cake

Angelic flavor, and devilishly delicious. This is a carnivore version of angel cake and it is guaranteed to leave you satisfied without any guilt. It contains only two main ingredients and is packed with protein. A zero-carb and carnivore-friendly delight for those who would like to please their sweet tooth.

Time: 35 minutes

Serving Size: 1 serving

Prep Time: 10 minutes

Cook Time: 20-25 minutes

Nutritional Facts/Info:

Calories: 128

Carbs: 4.2 g

Fat: 9.3 g

Protein: 9.3 g

Ingredients:

- 5 egg whites
- ¼ tsp cream of tartar
- **⅛ cup egg white protein powder**
- stevia to taste
- cinnamon to taste

Directions:

1. Preheat the oven to 375°F degrees.
2. Measure the egg whites and place in a dry bowl or a stand mixer.
3. Add the cream of tartar and whip the egg whites until they form stiff peaks.
4. Gently fold in the protein powder, stevia, and cinnamon. Make sure you do not add too much stevia or the sweetness could be a little bit overwhelming.
5. Grease a baking dish with butter or tallow.
6. Spoon the fluffed egg white mixture onto a baking dish of your choice and form into a cake shape.
7. Bake in the oven for 20-25 minutes until it is golden on top.

8. Enjoy as a snack or dessert.

Parmesan Tuna Patties

Not entirely sure what to do with tuna? Well, these tuna-Parm patties are a delicious alternative to merely dropping a scoop of tuna on your plate. It is delicious and low-carb so that you can enjoy it guilt-free. Any recipe that takes under 15 minutes to make is a winner. You can even store them in the fridge for a snack or as a grab-and-go meal.

Time: 15 minutes

Serving Size: 4 servings

Prep Time: 5 minutes

Cook Time: 10 minutes

Nutritional Facts/Info:

Calories: 105.4

Carbs: 1.8 g

Fat: 4.6 g

Protein: 13.8 g

Ingredients:

- 1 can of tuna (6 oz)
- 1 tbsp reduced fat/sugar mayonnaise
- 1 large egg
- 2 tbsp Parmesan cheese (finely grated)
- 2 tbsp ground flax meal
- ½ tsp garlic powder
- ½ tsp onion powder
- ½ tsp salt

Directions:

1. Drain the tuna until most of the excess water is removed.
2. Mix all of the ingredients together in a medium-sized bowl and form into patties using your hands. You can use about ¼ cup of the mixture per patty.
3. Grease a skillet with cooking spray and place it on medium-high heat. Place the patties in the skillet.
4. Once in the skillet, lightly press down with a fork to set each patty. Fry each one for a few minutes on each side until they appear brown on the edges. Flip them over and do the same on the other side. They should fry rather quickly.
5. Remove them from the skillet and let them rest for a few minutes before serving. Make sure

they are completely cooled before storing them in the fridge.

Condiments

Fish Sauce

Fish sauce is made only from sea salt and anchovies, but it provides a tasty umami flavor. As with many other condiments, it is recommended to double-check the ingredients label and be on the lookout for hidden sugars and carbohydrates. You can add it to chicken to give it some flavor, toss it in with some stir fried beef, add it to fish (obviously), and to eggs for that something extra.

Butter

Unlike other diets and weight-loss eating plans, the carnivore diet encourages the use of butter as a condiment. Butter can be consumed in slices, spread over meat, mixed into ground beef, or melted and drizzled onto your food. Butter is high in animal fat and is also a great way to grease pans, pots, skillets, grills, and other utensils. If you are sensitive to dairy, then you can substitute with ghee. It is not that hard to find and once you do, you will see its worth. Try using organic or raw local butter.

Reduction Sauce

Reduction sauce is a very dense sauce made from meat stock. Chicken stock or drippings from a roast can also be used. You can trim the fat off and save it for another use, let the remaining liquid simmer over medium-low heat until it becomes thick, and then add salt after the desired consistency is reached. Pour this reduction over sliced meat, chicken, or some liver for an extra-rich taste. To make it extra nutritious, you can also add in some bone marrow.

Baconnaise

You can make your own mayonnaise by using leftover bacon grease and some egg yolks. It goes great with eggs, salads, steaks, and chicken. The tangy taste is great if you are in the mood for a condiment that is not as dense as some other stocks and sauces. Just make sure you stay away from commercial mayonnaise because most of it contains sugar and other unwanted ingredients.

Homemade Sour Cream

Homemade sour cream contains beneficial probiotics and can be made from the type of cream or milk that you prefer. This means that you have complete control over the ingredients. Sour cream adds flavor and soupiness to any carnivore meal. If you have problems with lactose, keep in mind that homemade sour cream is much lower in lactose than dairy milk or even yogurt.

It is also a great way to liven up some recipes for the summer.

*Meat Marinades

Teriyaki Marinade: ¼ cup soy, ¼ cup maple syrup, ½ cup olive oil, 2 cloves garlic, 1 tsp ground ginger, 1 pinch of pepper, 1 tsp buckwheat flour.

Cilantro and Lime Marinade: 2 tbsp olive oil, 2 tbsp lime juice, ¼ cup cilantro, 1 tsp sea salt, and ground black pepper.

Basil and Balsamic Marinade: 3 tbsp balsamic vinegar, ¼ cup olive oil, 1 tbsp dried basil, 1 tsp sea salt, 2 cloves garlic.

Hawaiian Marinade: ½ cup pineapple juice, 3 tbsp soy sauce, 2 tbsp olive oil, ½ tsp onion powder, ½ tsp dried ginger, 1 tsp sea salt, and ground black pepper.

Fajita Marinade: ¼ cup olive oil, ¼ cup maple syrup, ½ tsp chili powder, ¼ tsp cumin powder, ½ tsp paprika, 1 tsp onion powder, 1 tsp garlic powder, 2 tbsp lime juice.

BBQ Marinade: ½ cup reduced sugar barbeque sauce, ¼ cup maple syrup, ¼ cup apple cider vinegar, ½ tbsp chili powder.

*Keep in mind that these marinades can be used occasionally and it is recommended that the low number of carbohydrates from them are suitable for the carnivore diet.

Chapter 6:

A Week in the Life of a Carnivore

This chapter will provide you with a sample 2-week meal plan that you can refer to for guidance when planning your own meals. It is structured for each day to have 2 meals to be adjusted as needed so that you are satiated and energized throughout the day. At the end of the chapter, you find some basic kitchen items and seasoning that will be useful to keep on hand. The cooking styles in the meal plan are recommendations, but you should feel comfortable to use whatever preparation method you prefer. As time goes on your meals and preparations will become second nature. Basically, all you have to do is get into the flow and you will do great, remember to give yourself enough time to get into the swing of things and do not overwhelm yourself with unnecessary stress. Stick to what you are used to in Level 1 and then start experimenting in Level 2. It is all worth it in the end.

Because of our busy schedules we barely find some time in the day to do all the things that we want to do. Sure, it is possible to meet certain expectations and execute certain tasks during the day, but that could leave you feeling tired, drained, and apathetic from time to time. There might not be enough time to shop, let alone cook, and that is why we want to grab the fastest and easiest meals we can find. Whether it's just a nibble or an entire meal, we often grab and run, without paying much attention to the nutrients or ingredients that we are consuming. This is also why we tend to order take out or indulge in fast food rather than spend time at the stove. These fast foods and quick fixes can be very unhealthy and are some of the predominant drivers behind weight gain and health issues.

Meal preparation and menu planning is considered to be a strategically beneficial method to aid in your weight loss, sustain a balanced lifestyle, and to become more organized without the added pressures that come with following a special eating pattern. Meal prep and planning is not difficult to adjust as you please and modify according to your schedule and preferences. Luckily, you do not have to be an expert planner to find success during your carnivore diet journey; you just have to adapt to the idea of strategizing. Making a list of the things you need before shopping will significantly decrease your chances of overspending or succumbing to the urge of buying fast food as a quick fix. For example, you can do a weekly shopping trip and use these items to prepare your meals for the week ahead. Saving your leftovers and working them into your menu for the next day is also a great way to save some time.

There are many great options for meal prepping and planning, and it is really something that you can customize and adjust to your own home life and schedule.

The recommended approach to this way of insightful eating and shopping is to think about your environment. If you are cooking for one, you will certainly have less prepping and shopping to do, whereas cooking for a household can become tremendously pressured. When you are catering for a bunch of people, it is simpler to prepare meals for about two or more days. When prepping for one person, you can do two to three days or even just heat up and eat the leftovers the next day. It is wise to store your food pre-cooked for no longer than five days in the fridge. That is why it could be helpful to work out a menu in advance that will help you to get into the flow of meal prepping and planning. When you are following the carnivore diet, you will notice that it requires a lot of cooking, so meal prepping and planning can make your experience less stressful or tedious.

Planning and preparing your food in advance has a lot of advantageous aspects to it. It benefits you financially and defeats the need to spend money on take-out lunches or fast food. It also has a very significant effect on weight loss or maintenance because it gives you control over the ingredients that you use and the serving portions eaten. This also amounts to less food waste and in the long run, provides you with more nutrients and sustainability. In many ways, it can also lessen certain forms of stress and anxiety because you do not have to be concerned about last minute cooking or food preparation. When you have extra time on your hands, you may even feel more motivated to exercise or partake in physical activities that will improve your physical and mental health overall.

When you start your prepping, it is always recommended to try some form of multitasking. It can be helpful to cook something on the stove while you are preparing something in the oven, for example. As you start doing this often, you will steadily become accustomed to the order in which these things are done and what caters best to your needs. No one is skilled enough to figure it out at the first try, but as you go on to do this, you will soon get the hang of it. Like most things, it becomes simpler and easier over time. When it comes to flavoring certain foods, you can even do it during the previous day or night, even if it is on the menu for the following day. It will free up some of your preparation time and give you some extra time to focus on your cooking.

Here is a valuable tip for storing your pre-cooked meals. The best way is to let them cool down completely before storing them. This will guarantee that your food does not spoil while it is in the fridge. Using see-through or transparent containers for storage will help you to determine when and how to plan your meals and makes it easier to see what you are taking from the fridge without opening up and peeking inside every container. Marking or adding labels to your containers with dates, descriptions, and/or icons may also make it easier to identify what is stored inside.

Tips for Meal Planning

1. Make a well-thought-out menu. Choose which recipes you will make for lunch and dinner and make a list of the items that you will need from the grocery store or market. When you have a set plan, you will be reluctant to spend money on fast food or unhealthy snacks.
2. Plan your meals around promotions and sales. Check your local grocery store for flyers, newspaper inserts, and coupons. Nowadays, you can even go online and seek out specials for certain items, so do take advantage of that. It will make your journey easier and more affordable. Even though certain foods may be on promotion or sale, do not buy foods that are not on your menu/list. They can go to waste or mess with your plans.
3. Plan at least 3 or 4 meals per week that contain eggs. Eggs offer great-tasting protein at a very low cost. Eggs will also make you feel fuller longer, which makes for a great meat substitute.
4. Double-check your pantry, refrigerator, and freezer often. Look at the expiry dates on the foods and ingredients that you have on hand. Use the ones that are due to expire first. In this way, you will not get stuck throwing out expensive animal products.

5. Stay away from recipes that need special ingredients. There are recipes available that require a special, one-of ingredient that you may not have. If you are adamant to follow this recipe and if you feel like it is worth it, then feel free to make the purchase. A good way to handle this is to substitute with ingredients that you have on hand. This will save you effort, time, and money.
6. Use your leftovers. Incorporate the previous night's dinner into your menu for the next morning or afternoon. If you store your leftovers efficiently and safely, you can utilize them for approximately two days after initial preparation. For example, if you are making roast beef for Sunday night's supper, then you can make a beef and egg omelet the next morning or for lunch. On Tuesday, use the bones to make a broth.
7. Make extras. Use it all by preparing a big pot of soup or a nice stew. If ground beef is on sale, make two batches of meat lasagna instead of one. Eat one batch for dinner and freeze the rest in portions for the next day or week.
8. Get familiar with what others in the house like to eat. Inspire your household to share their favorites and help with meal planning. In this way, everyone can take turns with cooking,

sharing, or just keeping an eye out for specials and promotions.
9. You will probably experience fatigue, headaches, and other flu-like symptoms during the first few days of the diet. It is extremely important to push through this stage because it gets easier with time. DO NOT QUIT! You will also likely lose some weight, but just because you are making progress, do not get too comfortable. Plateaus are normal, and quitting before you have completed all of the levels regardless of how much weight you've lost or improvements you've made is ill-advised. Quitting too soon will cause weight regain over time and all your trouble and effort will be for nothing. Remember, it is a marathon and not a sprint.
10. Keep in mind that your appetite will fluctuate. You will experience some moments or days where you either constantly want to eat or snack or perhaps you will not have much of an appetite at all. This will also stabilize once you have adjusted to the diet, so do not worry. If you do not cheat on the bad days, then stabilization will occur even faster. It is important to make sure that your diet includes enough fat as well as protein, so fatty cuts of meat and fatty fish are encouraged. If you are

constantly hungry, you may need to add more fat into your meal rotations.

Frequently Asked Questions:

Does it work for athletes and avid exercisers?

Yes. Many fitness buffs assume that glucose from carbs is the best source for quick and immediate energy. Your body will go through a process called gluconeogenesis where some protein is turned into glucose to be used for certain body functions.

Is processed meat allowed?

It is important to remember that processed meat like sandwich meat, pepperoni, etc. is often packed with toxins and unidentifiable ingredients. It is not exactly safe and in this case, organic is always better.

How long does it take to adapt?

A few weeks to a month. You have most likely been consuming carbohydrates your whole life. Due to the role that carbohydrates have played in your diet over the years, you will realize that it takes a while to get used to this way of eating. Once the first few weeks have passed, then you will be 100% in the game.

How much meat should I eat daily when I am following the carnivore diet?

The carnivore diet is not a calorie-restrictive diet because of the fact that you already have to cut so many carbohydrates from your diet. That is why you are free to eat as many calories as you need to. It is a diet designed to remove inflammatory foods and other ingredients that modern nutrition has introduced (Phelps, 2020). All you have to do is eat until you are full. Listen to your body.

Will my body go into ketosis?

The carnivore diet aims for low or zero-carbs, so naturally your system will begin to choose to burn fat over carbs and sugar.

Will I build muscle on the carnivore diet?

Due to an increase in average protein intake, you are likely to build muscle mass. If you are interested in becoming fairly muscular, then adding some carnivore-approved supplements will definitely help you to reach your goal.

Below, you will find a great example of a two-week carnivore meal plan. You can use this as a guide to structuring your own meals. As you can see, some meals are repeated every other day. This will help you to utilize your leftovers and save some time, money, and effort. It is important to remember that each person is different, so if you find that eating only two meals a day is not working for you, then stick to three. You can also use some of the snack recipes in Chapter 5 to quell hunger pangs between meals. Whatever you do, just be sure that you stay full and hydrated. If your body is nourished regularly, then you will notice how much less your brain will obsess about eating and even cheating. It is common for people to cheat on their diets when they are not eating enough or staying hydrated.

Week 1

Day 1,4

- Breakfast - Roasted salmon with seasoning
- Dinner - Grilled lamb chops

Day 2,5

- Breakfast - Ribeye steak
- Dinner - Ground beef patty

Day 3,6

- Breakfast - Bone marrow
- Dinner - Roasted pork belly

Day 7

- Breakfast - Cod fillets
- Dinner - Slow cooked chuck roast

Week 2

Day 8,11

- Lunch - Ribs with tallow
- Dinner - Beef patty

Day 9,12

- Lunch - Seared ribeye steak
- Dinner - Pork chops

Day 10,13

- Lunch - Grilled salmon fillets
- Dinner - Lamb burgers

Day 14

- Lunch - Roasted pork belly
- Dinner - Roasted shrimp and ribeye

Remember to add some variety to your meal plan and to switch it up every other week with new recipes or with something you have never tried before. Add some eggs in the beginning of your carnivore journey and then, slowly but surely, lessen the amount of eggs that you consume. Do not try to cut everything out from day 1. This is not a quick and easy fix, so the chances of you relapsing and going back to old habits will be more likely if you go about it too fast. It takes time, patience, effort, and commitment. Keep in mind that your body will change moderately and slow progress does not mean failure.

Carnivore Shopping List

MEAT
- Beef Steaks
- Beef Roasts
- Ground Beef (NOT lean)
- Lamb Chops
- Ground Lamb
- Ground Bison
- Pork Belly
- Pork Chops
- Bacon
- Roast Chicken
- Chicken Thigh
- Chicken Wings
- Ground Chicken
- Wild Game
- Venison
- Beef Liver
- Chicken Liver
- Bison Liver

SEAFOOD

- Fresh Salmon
- Canned Salmon
- Canned Sardines
- Canned Mackerel
- Canned Anchovies
- Canned Cod Liver
- Canned Tuna
- Shrimp
- Oysters
- Crab
- Lobster
- Canned Mussels

FAT

- Butter
- Ghee
- Beef Tallow
- Bison Tallow
- Lard
- Beef Suet
- Duck Fat
- Chicken Fat
- Bone Marrow
- Any other animal fat

ADD-ONS

- Chicken Eggs
- Duck Eggs

- Bone Broth
- Collagen Powder
- Pork Rinds
- Beef Jerky
- Aged Cheeses
- Kefir
- Full Fat Yoghurt
- Sour Cream
- Heavy Cream
- Raw Milk

SPICES and HERBS
- White Pepper
- Garlic
- Onion Powder
- Ginger
- Dill
- Basil
- Rosemary
- Thyme
- Chives
- Cilantro
- Parsley
- Sage
- Cinnamon
- Vanilla

OTHER

- Salt
- Magnesium (Capsules, Powders)
- Electrolyte Powder
- Beef Liver Capsules
- Cod Liver Oil
- Krill Oil

Stocking your kitchen

In order for you to successfully prepare all of these delicious meals, in addition to high-quality ingredients, you need access to the correct utensils and supplies. It will make your life and your carnivore journey a lot easier to maintain if you use the correct tools in the kitchen. Investing in a good all-purpose knife, for example, will save time and meal prep will not be as tedious in the long run. If you use the wrong knife, you might end up with a mess in the kitchen or injuring yourself. There are a lot of good options online.

Here is a list of things that might come in handy:

Meat thermometer: No one likes their meat to be overcooked. This thermometer will prevent you from undercooking or overcooking your meat. It measures the internal temperature which will help you to determine where your meat is, based on the cooking scale. If you are one of those cooks who tends to overcook your meat beyond dry, then this is ideal.

Ziplock and freezer bags: These little plastic bags are great for storing leftover meat in the freezer. It is also a great way to monitor what and how much you have left.

Pots and pans: You will find that having durable, high-quality, non-stick pots and pans are a must with any diet. It saves you a lot of scrubbing time and you do not have to compensate by greasing. They will also cook meat more evenly to your satisfaction.

Slow/pressure cooker: They are great for stews, roasts, soups, broths, and many other dishes. They also make your cooking experience less daunting because they do all the work for you. Investing in one of these is a must.

A good knife set: Knives, cleavers, boning knives, etc. are essential when you are working with meat. You do not want to spend all this time, money, and effort on the perfect meal just to ruin your meat cuts by using cheap or unsuitable knives. You can also do some research on how to use them correctly so that you know exactly how to invest.

Meat mallet or heavy rolling pin: There will be times when a thin cutlet, breaded and quickly fried is all you crave and in this case, a meat mallet or heavy rolling pin is the only tool you will need to prepare your dish. It also comes in handy when you are in the mood to tenderize before cooking.

Solid wooden cutting board: Wooden cutting boards (the thick and sturdy kind) are great for preparing proteins. There will be minimal staining and damage to your kitchen counters, and it simplifies the cooking experience immensely.

Supplements for Carnivores

The carnivore diet takes on a rather restrictive approach which inevitably can source out some of the dangers of nutrient deficiencies and digestive issues. Your protein consumption will certainly not be deficient from all of the beef consumption, but if you overlook certain micronutrients and cut out salt for long enough, you can start to feel generally depraved and even experience some more serious health issues.

Magnesium

Sadly, most meat does not contain high quantities of magnesium, and even when consuming several pounds of meat daily, you can develop deficiencies over time.

There are certain health risks that can occur when you develop a magnesium deficiency. Magnesium is one of the most vital minerals that your body requires. It is sourced for numerous distinct functions that, within a few months of deficiency, can lead to considerable health issues. Your metabolism needs it to utilize energy, it plays a role in controlling hormone levels, your muscles need it to produce protein, and it is still essential for DNA production (Woods, 2020). One of your choices is to eat fish eggs on a regular basis or to make your own beef bone broth using a slow cooking method. Instead, you can get extra magnesium from taking an Epsom salt bath. However, it is best to purchase magnesium supplements from your local pharmacy or store. Deficiencies can become a big obstacle in your journey, and it is always best to be safe.

Potassium

Potassium is another important nutrient and, as an electrolyte, it plays a dynamic role in the fluid balance in all your body's cells. Generally, meat is not a great supplier of potassium, except if you frequently consume organ meats. A deficiency of potassium on a regular basis can lead to an upsurge in blood pressure, possible kidney stones, deteriorated muscle function, and even abnormal or erratic heart rates. With the risk of heart disease commonly on the rise, electrolyte shortcomings such as this have to be carefully observed.

Vitamin C and E

Vitamin C is an essential nutrient that we must consume with our food because our body cannot produce it from other sources or nutrients. It is most commonly found in plant foods like fruits. Animal foods do not have it in abundance and unfortunately, most meats and animal products do not really contain vitamin C at all. You can boost your vitamin levels by eating more organ meats like the spleen or the lung. It might sound a bit unappetizing, so you might want to opt for supplements instead. Vitamin E deficiency is more common in carnivores who do not eat organic or grass-fed meat. Eating cheaper alternatives, like grain-fed meat, tends to cause your vitamin E levels to drop considerably which is not a desirable side effect (Woods, 2020).

Fiber

One thing you will struggle to find in most meats is fiber. It is one of the key drawbacks of shifting to a carnivore lifestyle, but the tangible health benefits are unclear. On the one side, high fiber carbohydrates are viewed as an integral part of a fat-loss diet because they keep you full and keep your digestion from slowing down. There is no wrong or right way to approach the claim that a carnivore diet causes a lack of fiber in the body.

It is important to remember that all bodies are different and, if you do feel like your digestion has slowed down a bit, you can supplement your fiber intake. There are thousands of fiber supplement products on the market and you can use them in the morning when your metabolism needs a boost the most. Be sure to use natural and safe fiber supplements to avoid side effects like diarrhea, dehydration, and water retention.

Ketones

The carnivore lifestyle or diet is often referred to as the keto diet in overdrive (Woods, 2020). As you already know by now, you will mainly be eating high-fat and high-protein foods from mostly beef in the long run. This includes avoiding carbohydrates derived from plant foods and dairy products including yogurt, milk, and cheese, which are only an option for you in the beginning stages of the diet because eventually, you will have to cut them out completely.

Early on in your journey, before ketosis has set in, you will still be adaptable to the fat intake. This is when you will likely experience the worst side effects of the "keto-flu" which contains side effects like headaches, nausea, low energy levels, and overall discomfort. After a few days, these side effects will begin to subside as your body adjusts. When your body starts to produce ketones for energy, you will experience a noticeable amount of fat loss. Your body will then be in ketosis which is fat-burning for the energy phase.

According to Woods (2020), these are not extended effects and you will not experience this for very long which makes it easy to get through. However, your blood sugar levels can drop to a very low level, despite the fact that you are consuming enough protein and fat. You can either ride it out or take some ketone supplements to make the side effects a little bit more bearable. It is crucial to drink a lot of water during this experience and refrain from using caffeine as an energy source because it can make the sensation worse. Dehydration should not be taken lightly, and water retention will cause the scale to tip up a considerable amount.

Polyphenols

Polyphenols are not something you hear about often and they have only recently caught the attention of many carnivore diet experts. It is a plant-based group of antioxidants that has been studied through clinical trials. There are not a lot of scientific facts that have surfaced yet, but it seems like there might be a link between polyphenols and the protection against certain cancers and heart disease. Animal foods, like meat and eggs, do not contain any polyphenols, so your best option is to use supplements (Woods, 2020). It is not a mandatory supplement, but it might help to ease some fears or even help with certain feelings of discomfort throughout the adjustment period.

Collagen

Collagen supplements have gained popularity over the years, and the reasons for this are almost too obvious. Unfortunately, collagen is a nutrient that is mostly found in the parts of the animal that are not edible, unless you have an unethical way of dieting. It is mostly found in connective tissue and tendons, parts that are quite difficult to make edible (Woods, 2020).

It is a significant nutrient that promotes healthy skin, joints, connective tissue, and bones. It has also become an extremely sought after supplement in the carnivore diet. A lot of people claim to have seen changes in their skin, hair, joints, and muscles from consuming it. Collagen supplements can be consumed in many ways, like capsules, powders, oils, creamers, etc. Whichever preference you have, there is likely an option available for you.

Chapter 7:

Implementing the Carnivore Diet in Your Life

Transitioning to the carnivore lifestyle can be challenging for anyone, even those who are transitioning from paleo or ketogenic diets. It takes a lot of willpower and determination to make such big changes in your life. However difficult it may be, it is absolutely the best decision you can make. There are many people who have made this change and who can attest that their lives have changed significantly, in the best ways possible. They are experiencing no more underlying health problems, unwanted fat, fatigue, brain fog, etc. If you can picture yourself living a life that is happy, healthy, and rich in vitality, then you have already taken the first step. Below, you will find some crucial tips and advice that will help you to make this transition as smooth as possible.

Start small

Starting small can be useful when it comes to the carnivore diet. If you are coming from a rather unhealthy or carbohydrate-rich diet, then the change might be more difficult for you than someone who is coming from a low-carbohydrate diet. People who consume a lot of sugar also have a hard time due to sugar addiction and experiencing a detox similar to those who have problems with substance abuse. It sounds serious because it is. You may wish to address a possible sugar addiction before diving into the carnivore lifestyle, as the frightening thing is, there are millions of people who are unaware that they have this problem at all.

This does not mean that you have a definite sugar addiction, and in fact, it is quite normal to crave something sweet from time to time. Cravings occur for various reasons like low blood sugar, hormones, a lack of protein, dehydration, etc. Most people use sugar in unhealthy ways, even if it does not amount to addiction. If you tend to crave sugary treats and give into those cravings by binging on unhealthy foods, then it might be a bigger problem for you than others. According to (Ratini, 2020), sugar fuels cells in the brain and the brain also views it as a reward which is why you might keep craving it time after time. If you consume a lot of sugar, you are fortifying this notion, which then turns into a very unhealthy habit.

Have you ever wondered why you get a sugar rush or high after eating a treat during the day? This is because the sugar in that treat, also known as a simple carbohydrate, turns into glucose in the bloodstream quite rapidly. This causes your blood sugar levels to spike vigorously, leaving you hyperactive or tense for a brief moment. Simple carbs are also present in fruits, vegetables, and dairy products. However, these foods also contain fiber and protein which causes the process to slow down and glucose is distributed moderately (Ratini, 2020).

Your body has to move glucose from the bloodstream into your cells to generate energy and your pancreas produces insulin (a hormone) to make this process happen. This results in a sudden drop in your blood sugar levels which leaves you feeling tired, shaky, weak, and in the need for more sugar to regain your buzz or any energy at all (Ratini, 2020). You then go back to unhealthy treats to regain your energy and this eventually turns into a very unhealthy cycle and sugar dependency.

Even foods like bagels, chips, or French fries when consumed turn into sugars. These starchy foods are complex carbs that the body breaks down into simple sugars. Eaten without better foods, starches can make blood sugar surge and crash just like sugar. White rice and white flour do this. Highly refined starches like white bread, pretzels, crackers, and pasta are worse (Ratini, 2020). Sugar can be found in foods where you least expect it. They might not seem sweet, but ketchup, barbecue sauce, and pasta sauce can have loads of sugar. Frankly, most condiments contain sugar, even the ones who claim to be 'healthier' like reduced-fat salad dressings, bread, baked beans, and flavored coffees and teas. This is why the carnivore diet encourages the reading of ingredient labels of food before purchase.

Now that you are approaching a healthier way of life, it is important to know that you can teach your taste buds to enjoy things that are not high in sugar. Try cutting out one sugary treat or food from your diet daily. For example, pass on dessert after dinner and start putting less or no sugar at all in your coffee, tea, or cereal. You will realize that over time, you do not feel the need for sugar at all.

Protein will not make your blood sugar rise the way refined carbs and sugars do. The carnivore diet is also a great way out of your sugar obsession. Consuming protein is the best way to beat those sugar cravings. High-protein foods digest more slowly, which leaves you feeling satiated longer.

So, before you start thinking about reaching Level 1 of the carnivore diet, try to eliminate sugar from your daily diet first. It will make your adjustment phase easier and you will feel better overall. You can also take this time to educate yourself on the hidden sugars found in most of the 'healthy' foods that you were considering incorporating into your meal plan. It is best to stay away from store-bought sauces and rather make your own that use the same principles as the carnivore diet. Broths and marinades are easy to prepare at home and they taste amazing.

When it comes to cutting out plant-based carbohydrates like fruits, vegetables, grains, etc. from your diet, it can be quite difficult at first. It is not realistic nor sustainable to go full on cold turkey right from the start. Instead, you can start by cutting out fruits. Instead of grabbing a piece of fruit to snack on, try eating a few spoons of yoghurt or substitute it with a boiled egg.

Vegetables tend to be the hardest ones to cut out because so many people rely on the 'nutrients' that they contain. Once you have eliminated fruits from your diet, you can move onto only eating vegetables with your dinner twice a week. After a while, you will forget whatever was attracting you to them. The same goes with other carbohydrates, so try to eat them only every other day until you do not feel the need for them anymore.

Another essential thing to remember when you are starting your carnivore journey, is to not overwhelm yourself with difficult or time-consuming recipes at first. You will become better at preparing meals over time and it will become easier to follow recipes in due time. No one steps into this lifestyle and becomes an expert right away. Not only are you adjusting to eating differently, but you are also adjusting to cooking differently. Simple meals like hamburgers and steaks can be just as delicious and satisfying as hearty stews or broths, for example. Keep it simple in the beginning until you become better equipped to handle more complex meals.

Plan ahead

It is a lot easier to stick to a plan when you already know what your next meal is going to be. Dieting without meal planning takes a lot of time, effort, and patience and you will thank yourself if you learn how to incorporate meal prepping and planning into your weekly schedule. Dealing with work, socializing, family, and other activities can be exhausting and having to prepare a meal twice a day as well can take a chunk out of your day. Instead, set up a weekly menu that involves leftovers and meal preparation to ease the pressure a little bit. Grab and go meals are also possible on the carnivore diet, so there is no need to overwhelm yourself. If a full meal plan is too involved, start by planning one meal a day and increase it as you start to feel more comfortable.

Tailor your food to your preferences

Take advantage of seasonings, fats like butter, and different cooking styles. Scott Myslinski (Woods, 2020) advises to focus on the cuts of meat you find the most delicious and not to worry about organs at the start as you will not develop any nutrient deficiencies in 90 days. Many 10-plus-year carnivores do not eat organs at all. He also adds that you can always adjust the diet later on or as you become more comfortable, but if you are still skeptical you can check out some carnivore-approved supplements (Woods, 2020).

He also states that it is important to eat the required amount for you to feel full. Focus on your body and its needs, and do not overeat. Eat as much as you want and if it is necessary, eat often. Do not go into the diet expecting to lose weight immediately. If you do that and deprive yourself, you will not adapt to eating only meat and you will be much more likely to give in to cravings and fail (Woods, 2020).

Learn How to Differentiate Between Hunger and Thirst

Confusing your appetite for thirst is normal, and it is important to know the difference if you are aiming or trying to lose weight. Confusing these two strong cravings will lead you to eat more calories than you need and sabotage reaching your goals of weight loss. The same section of your brain is responsible for processing signs of hunger and thirst and can sometimes contribute to mixed messages. You should try to eat every three to four hours, and you may only be thirsty if you feel hungry between meals. If your normal liquid consumption starts with a few cups of coffee, you may already be dehydrated by the time you feel thirsty. Symptoms of dehydration include dry eyes, pain in the brain, sluggishness, nausea, and dizziness. There may also be dark yellow urine, and your mouth may feel dry. Drink water during the day at regular intervals, even if you do not feel thirsty, and you will have less risk of getting dehydrated (Corporate Wellness Magazine, n.d.).

A big part of carnivore success is the fact that you will be consuming a lot of water daily which will flush out toxins and keep you hydrated. If you are someone who tends to struggle with drinking water regularly, you may wish to try these ideas:

Set a goal. The suggested amount of water per day is half of your body weight in ounces. Once you know the amount, make it a challenge to get at least that set amount every day. Turn it into a water-drinking challenge with friends or family to remain motivated.

Set a timer for mental triggers. Create a few alarms on your phone, and each time they go off, you will be inclined to drink some water. You can also download a water-drinking app that has the same feature and a water counter as well. You will also see less fluid retention which can make a big difference on the scale.

Freeze some small pieces of fruit in place of ice cubes and try adding a little ginger. Bubbly or sparkling water is also tasty and provides hydration without the added sugar. This also helps you to stay away from sodas and other carbonated drinks that might be harmful to your health.

Always drink a lot of water before and after any type of exercise. By the time you actually realize that you are starting to feel a bit parched during a workout, your body is already on the path to dehydration and you may not have noticed. It is also good to fuel up on electrolyte supplements before workouts so that if you do not consume enough water during the activity, you will at least have something to make up for the lack of hydration.

Things to avoid

Do not consume fruits and vegetables at all during the first weeks of Level 3. One of the reasons this diet is so effective is because it induces ketosis, which requires no- or low-carbohydrate levels. Such consumption will take your body out of ketosis, stunt your progress, and you will have to kick-start the process all over again, which will waste a lot of your time and previous efforts.

Some people also make the mistake of buying or consuming too much lean meat. It is important to remember that fatty proteins will provide more energy and keep you full longer. If you do not consume enough fat, it will cause your energy levels to drop and your body could start storing fat in order to prepare itself for some sort of shutdown. Organic, grass-fed, and fatty meats are the best options.

Be patient

All diets take time, but the carnivore diet requires particular patience because your body will take time to adjust to this new ratio of fat/protein to carbs. Something as sustainable and effective as the carnivore diet will take a bit more time than some random calorie-restricted crash diet, but the benefits are more permanent, especially when it comes to health and weight loss. It is not like you cannot enjoy a sneaky cheat every now and then, so there really is no reason to experience the fear of missing out. You just have to teach yourself how to cheat in moderation.

Eating out

While your choices at restaurants will be quite obvious, you will often find yourself in a sticky situation where you have to explain or justify your dietary choices. Dr. Shawn Baker (Woods, 2020) states that you should realize that you are eating for your health and for your own interest. You do not need to apologize, or feel ashamed, for what you are eating. People who are critical about what you are eating are not going to pay your medical bills when your health is affected.

When you are having dinner, or any other meal time with friends for example, you may order something like meat only without any carbs and this might raise some eyebrows. Be prepared to answer and inform those around you. You do not have to be disrespectful, but it helps to be well educated on the topic and its opposition. By welcoming and answering questions informatively, you just might encourage friends and family to try it for themselves too. Respond naturally to comments, and state that you're making your own health choices and aren't pushing them on anyone else (Woods, 2020).

Remember that you are doing this for your own health and no one else's. You have the chance and the opportunity to regain control of your health and your life. Do not let someone take that chance away from you just because they disagree or dislike the way you have decided to live. When you feel like you have to explain yourself constantly, you will lose confidence in the process. If someone is rude to you about it, you should simply shrug it off and keep your end goal in mind. Perhaps use this opportunity to prove them wrong.

Chapter 8:

The Nutritional Value of Meat

According to Ahmad et al. (2018, p. 2169), meat is high among the most substantial, nutritious and energy-rich natural food products consumed by humans to fulfill their regular body and mind requirements. It is considered crucial in the act of maintaining a healthy and balanced diet, something that is vital in achieving optimum human growth and development. Its role in the human species' evolution, specifically in our brains and intellectual development, cannot be ignored. According to the European Legislation (Ahmad et al. 2018, p. 2169), meat is termed as the portions obtained from domestic animals including caprine, bovine, ovine, and porcine, also including poultry meat, and farmed and wild animals that are edible. It is arguably the main supplier of high-value proteins, a variety of fats like zinc, iron, selenium, potassium, magnesium, sodium, vitamin A, B-complex vitamins, folic acid, and Omega-3 polyunsaturated fatty acids.

From a nutritional outlook, meat is considered an integral essential amino acid source whereas minerals tend to have a less significant impact. Not only that, but meat also is also a source of essential fatty acids and vitamins. Organ meats like liver are a highly enriched source of Vitamin A, Vitamin B1, and nicotinic acid. The research is still inconclusive regarding a better understanding of the apparent differences among the nutritional assessment of different meat cuts, animal species and breeds (Ahmad et al., 2018, p. 2169). It is evident from previous research that meat containing only small amounts, or no connective tissue, is likely to have fewer signs of required digestion and absorption. In addition, the meat containing more connective tissues is supposed to have fewer essential amino acids, which make it less nutritious in comparison to the meat containing less connective tissue and results in more digestibility and nutritional content (Ahmad et al. 2018, p.2169).

Meat cut	Protein (g)	Sat. fat (g)	Fat (g)	Energy (kcal)	Vit. B_{12} (mcg)	Na (mg)	Zn (mg)	P (mg)	Fe (mg)
Chicken breast, raw	24.2	0.2	8.5	178	0.39	71	0.9	199	1.2

Beef, steak cuts, raw	21	1.9	4.5	123	1.9	59	1.7	16.7	1.3
Chicken, raw	22.8	0.6	1.9	113	0.70	78	1.4	20.2	0.7
Beef, calf, loin, raw	20	3.4	7.3	146	1.1	22	3	19.3	0.110
Beef, loin, raw	20.9	1.5	3.2	115	2	59	3.7	14.2	1.6
Pork, chop, raw	18.1	10.8	31.7	353	1	60	1.8	19.0	1.4
Pork, loin, raw	21.9	1.7	4.9	134	1.1	55	1.9	22.0	0.7

Pork, leg, raw	20.8	2.8	7.8	155	1.2	84	2.6	164	0.8
Turkey, skinless, raw	19.9	1.8	7.1	136	1.9	42	1.5	209	2.1
Duck meat, skinless, raw	19.4	1.8	6.6	130	2.8	90	1.8	201	2.5
Turkey, breast, skinless, raw	23.6	0.5	1.6	106	1	62	0.5	208	0.6
Chicken breast, skinless, raw	23.8	0.4	1.28	109	0.40	59	0.7	218	0.4

| Mutton, chop or meat, raw | 20 | 2.4 | 4.8 | 122 | 2 | 63 | 3.6 | 22 | 1.9 |

Water

Water is one of the important components of all food materials. Generally, there are three types of food products depending upon their moisture contents; perishable commodities (having more than 70% moisture content in them), non-perishable commodities (having around 50–60% moisture contents), and stable food materials (with less than 15% moisture) (Ahmad et al., 2018, p. 2169). The higher the water content of any food material, the lesser the chances of a long shelf life because micro-organisms have a greater chance to grow on them which limits their longevity (Ahmad et al., 2018, p. 2169). So, if you are wondering how much water is in your food, just glance at the expiration or sell-by date. Anything that lasts for weeks is most likely preserved in a way where its water is reduced and replaced with preservatives to make it last longer. If the shelf life of a certain food is between a day and a week, it will most likely have a higher water content.

Meat is among the most perishable food material, as it contains more than 70% water. Apart from a significantly shorter shelf life, the amount or density of moisture (water) in meat can be seen with the naked eye in its impact on the discoloration and texture, and often, its bland flavor of muscle tissues. The tissue from the abdominal part of an animal usually contains less moisture or water, which assumes the fact that if the animal is fatter, it will have a lower water content in its body and vice versa. Younger and leaner animals have around 72% moisture content in their bodies (Ahmad et al., 2018, p. 2169). This implies that fattier meats have a lower moisture density or amount of water and leaner meats have a higher moisture density or water count. The principles of the carnivore diet are to limit your intake of lean meats. Fattier meats will keep you fuller longer and regardless of the water count in meats, you should still try to drink as much water as possible.

The majority of moisture in meat tissues exists in an unregimented state (meaning that it is distributed randomly and can move around freely) within muscle fibers and only a small amount of it is found in the connective tissues. During the processing stages, such as curing and heat treatment and then the storage, a small amount of the water is retained inside of the muscle fiber which is also known as the "bound water" (Ahmad et al., 2018, p. 2169). The three-dimensional structure of muscle fiber stimulated with the pressure and temperature enables the water to be retained in the muscles during the processing stages, while the rest of the water that is discarded during these circumstances is known as "free water." The amount of water storage in meat may be altered by the disruptions of its muscle fibers, which contribute to the development of the longevity or decay of meat products. There are numerous methods involved in this regard including chopping, grinding, salting, freezing, thawing, breakdown of connective tissues by enzymatic or chemical means, heating application, and use of chemicals or organic additives altering the acidity (pH) of meat (Ahmad et al., 2018, p. 2169). It is always best to scout out meat products that are produced organically. Chemical compounds used during production can mess with both your health and weight.

Carbohydrates

Regardless of the fact that the carnivore diet is based on the principle of consuming little to no carbohydrates, there is still a small amount of carbs found in meat. According to Ahmad et al. (2018, p. 2169), the main source of carbohydrates in the animal's body is its liver, which contains about half of the total number of carbohydrates present in the body. They are stored as glycogen, largely in the liver and muscles, but also in glands and organs to a lesser extent. Larger amounts are present in the blood and take the form of glucose. The glycogen content does not have a direct impact on the meat color, texture, tenderness, or water density (Ahmad et al., 2018, p. 2169). The conversion of stored glycogen to glucose, and from glucose to lactic acid, is an intricate process and all these processes are controlled by the roles of hormones and enzymes (Ahmad et al., 2018, p. 2169). Therefore, the amount of edible carbohydrates found in meat is not really significant.

During the early stages of development, the lactic acid content of the muscles increases, which lowers the pH. The pH has a significant impact on the muscles' texture, tenderness, color, and also on its water density. A normal pH of the muscle is approximately around 5.6 (Ahmad et al., 2018, p. 2169). If an animal experiences severe stress or overexercise just before the time of slaughter and has a low chance of regaining its normal glycogen levels, then a small amount of glycogen will form to be converted into lactic acid causing an elevated pH (6.5) and as a result, meat muscles become dark, firm, and dry. This defect is not desired by retailers and consumers, due to its effects on sensorial and nutritional properties (Ahmad et al.2018, p. 2169). This is why it is important to purchase your meat from ethically-sourced butchers or stores because the amount of stress that the animal endures can impact the nutritional value of the meat it provides. The main goal of the carnivore diet is to retain nutrients from the meat that you consume, so this is rather important to keep in mind when you are shopping for meat products.

Proteins and Amino Acids

Meat is a protein-rich food, providing high nutritional value to the world's populations. Proteins are naturally occurring, intricate nitrogenous compounds that carry significant molecular mass consisting of carbon, hydrogen, oxygen, and nitrogen which is also one of the most important compounds needed by the human body. Some proteins are also composed of traces of phosphorus and sulfur in their centres. These all bond together chemically to form different types of individual proteins, with variable properties. These differ from one bodily tissue to another within the same living organism and also in the same type of tissue of different species. The proteins are a lot more intricate and complicated than the carbohydrates and fats from their constituents. The amounts or mass of protein components found in meat varies notably in different types of meats (Ahmad et al., 2018, p. 2169). In general, the average value of the protein in meat is about 22%, but it could range from a higher protein value of 34.5% in chicken breast to as low as 12.3% protein in duck meat. Ahmad et al. (2018, p. 2169) also states that protein digestibility-corrected amino acid scores (PDCAAS), which depict the digestibility of a protein, reveal that meat has an overall high score of 0.92 compared to other protein sources including lentils, pinto beans, peas, and chickpeas scoring only 0.57-0.71. He also points out that the quality of the protein is mainly directed around the availability of amino acids present, which settles the debate on which food source contains the most protein; plants or animals. Amino acids serve as the building blocks and foundation of proteins. The nutritional value of meat can vary greatly by the occurring or non-occurring presence of numerous amino acids. One hundred and ninety two of them are easily identifiable and only 20 are used to prepare the proteins. From these 20 amino acids, 8 are viewed as the essential amino acids, as these could not be produced by the human body on its own, so they must be incorporated into the diet (Ahmad et al., 2018, p. 2169).The remaining 12 are the non-essential amino acids that could be produced by the human body, but only if certain food sources are being consumed, as if not consumed, it could result in protein malnutrition or deficiency (Ahmad et al., 2018, p. 2169). The table below shows the essential and non-essential amino acids found in meat:

Essential amino acids				
Amino acids	Category	Beef	Lamb	Pork
Lysine	Essential	8.2	7.5	7.9
Leucine	Essential	8.5	7.2	7.6
Isoleucine	Essential	5.0	4.7	4.8
Cystine	Essential	1.5	1.5	1.2
Threonine	Essential	4.2	4.8	5.2

Amino acid	Category	Beef	Lamb	Pork
Methionine	Essential	2.2	2.4	2.6
Tryptophan	Essential	1.3	1.2	1.5
Phenylalanine	Essential	4.1	3.8	4.3
Arginine	Essential	6.4	6.8	6.6
Histidine	Essential	2.8	2.9	3.1
Valine	Essential	5.6	5.1	5.2

Non-essential amino acids

Amino acid	Category	Beef	Lamb	Pork
Proline	Non-essential	5.2	4.7	4.4

Glutamic acid	Non-essential	14.3	14.5	14.6
Aspartic acid	Non-essential	8.9	8.6	8.8
Glycine	Non-essential	7.2	6.8	6.0
Tyrosine	Non-essential	3.3	3.3	3.1
Serine	Non-essential	3.9	3.8	4.1
Alanine	Non-essential	6.3	6.2	6.4

Beef has a higher amount of valine, lysine, and leucine when compared to lamb and pork. Studies have shown that the main reasoning behind these ratios of essential amino acids is based on the proportion within the breed, age, and muscle allocation. Research done beforehand included studies that concluded that the content of valine, isoleucine, phenylalanine, arginine and methionine in the meat becomes more prevalent as the meat or animal ageskick-start The essential amino acid contents also differ in the different parts of the carcass (Ahmad et al., 2018, p. 2169). They can also be compromised by processing techniques including heat and ionization radiations, but this only occurs when prolonged processes are being applied. In some cases, these amino acids are not made available for human consumption. Ahmad et al. (2018, p. 216) also states that another study showed that researchers discovered that only 50% of lysine was available at 160°C, while 90% of it was there at 70°C. Occasionally, the interaction between other constituents with the same proteins affects the progression of these amino acids. When a smoking and/or salting process is applied to the meat, it also affects the amount of essential amino acids that is being produced. Apart from the effect of the processing conditions, the storage has also imparted its effect on amino acids, in the case of canned meat (Ahmad et al., 2018, p. 2169).

Fat and Fatty Acids

Fat is viewed as one of the three top essential macronutrients, including carbohydrates and proteins. Fat structures are known as triglycerides that are components of three fatty acid links and the alcohol glycerol. Meat contains fatty tissues that do not all contain the exact same amounts of fat. In meat, fat content acts as energy deposits, a protective padding in the skin and around the organs like the heart and kidney. It also provides insulation against body temperature losses. Fat content in an animal carcass varies from 8% to 20% with the only difference found in pork (Ahmad et al., 2018, p. 2169). The fatty acid and fat composition of fatty tissue changes significantly in different locations of the body among poultry and other meat products such as offal, sausages, ham, etc. External body fat is softer than the internal fat that is layered around the organs. A higher amount of unsaturated fat is largely found in the external parts of the animal's body. Skin is the main source of fat in poultry meat. The meat cuts that are found in stores, like in chicken and turkey, ranges between 1% and 15% and meat cuts with the skin attached have a higher percentage (Ahmad et al., 2018, p. 2169). Cooking methods can have direct impacts on fatty acid composition found in the meat and meat fat content as well. Scientific evidence reported that considerable losses of fat in numerous meat cuts occurred during broiling, grilling, and pan-frying without added fat (Ahmad et al., 2018, p. 2169). Considering the importance of fat in the carnivore diet, you should always consider your cooking methods and the added fat that you use.

According to Ahmad et al. (2018, p. 2169), among the fatty acid composition, meat contains unsaturated fatty acids; oleic (C-18:1), linoleic (C-18:2), linolenic (C-18:3), and arachidonic (C-20:4) acid appear to be essential. They are extremely important inhibitors of the mitochondria which can be defined as the cell walls and other active metabolic sites. Linoleic acid (C-18:2) is also found in vegetable oils such as soya and corn oils, although its concentration is 20 times higher in meat and linolenic acid (C-18:3). Eicosapentaenoic acid (C-20:5) and docosahexaenoic acid (C-22:6) are normally found at low concentration in meat tissues, but it is also present at high concentrations in fish and fish oils (Ahmad et al., 2018, p. 2169). Polyunsaturated fatty acids, as well as the cholesterol in muscular and offal tissues of common edible meat species, are shown in the table below:

Meat source	Cholesterol (mg/100 g)	C-18:2	C-18:3	C-20:3	C-20:4	C-22:5	C-22:6
Mutton	81	2.4	2.4	Nil	Nil	Trace	Nil
Beef	62	2.1	1.4	Trace	1.1	Trace	Nil
Pork	71	7.5	1.0	Nil	Trace	Trace	1.1
Brain	2200	0.5	Nil	1.6	4.1	3.5	0.4

Pig's Kidney	415	11.6	0.4	0.5	6.72	Trace	Nil
Sheep's Kidney	399	8.2	4.1	0.6	7.2	Trace	Nil
Ox's kidney	401	4.9	0.6	Trace	2.7	Nil	Nil
Sheep's Liver	429	5.1	3.9	0.7	5.2	3.1	2.3
Pig's Liver	262	14.8	0.4	1.2	14.4	2.4	3.9

| Ox's Liver | 271 | 7.5 | 2.4 | 4.5 | 6.5 | 5.4 | 1.3 |

This table by Ahmad et al. (2018, p. 2169) shows that the linoleic acid concentration is more prominent in the lean meat of a pig than in ox or sheep's meat. These variations in the levels of fatty acids composition among different species are also revealed in kidney and liver fatty acid profiles. The liver tissue in all of these animal species is suggested as a vital product and a rich source of polyunsaturated fatty acids (Ahmad et al., 2018, p. 2169). On the other hand, the brain has a noticeably high concentration of C-22 polyunsaturated fatty acids that is produced regularly. It is tabulated that the concentration of cholesterol in offal tissues, particularly the brain, is more than the concentration in muscle tissues (Ahmad et al., 2018, p. 2169). Seeing that the brain is not the most appetizing part of the animal, even if it is the most nutritious, it is not expected of you to try it or incorporate it into your diet. However, it is important to recognize the benefits of each animal product and evaluate them before discarding the possibility (Ahmad et al., 2018, p. 2169). If you are not someone who tends to enjoy eating organs, you can slowly and surely introduce them into your diet by cooking them according to your own preferences.

Out of all the various polyunsaturated fatty acids, Omega-3 fatty acids are highly regarded and sought after because they play a protective and defining role in overall human health, and it stands out as a protection against cardiovascular disease. Seafood is the main edible source of Omega-3 fatty acids that comes from animal products, although meat can contribute up to 20% of the long chain Omega-3 polyunsaturated fatty acids (Ahmad et al., 2018, p. 2169). This polyunsaturated Omega-3 content in meat depends on how and what the animal is fed during its lifetime and it is considerably higher in animals that have a more organic or grass-fed diet. It is also suggested that polyunsaturated fatty acids found in animal fat are extremely important for the overall development of the brain, particularly in the fetus and its development. The chain extension of linoleic acid gives the prostaglandins a boost which is very important for regulating blood pressure. Prostaglandins are mostly found in organ meat and tissues and produced or conceived in the cell with the help of essential fatty acids. They are produced by all nucleated cells and are known as autocrine and paracrine lipid mediators that act on endothelium, uterine, and platelet cells (Ahmad et al., 2018, p. 2169).

A higher propensity for unsaturation in their fats and fatty tissues must be implemented in order to prevent possible adverse health effects from the consumption of ruminant animal meat. Generally, because of the reduction or condensation of rumen bacteria, the feeding of vegetable fats to sheep and cattle will be nullified. However, if they were first treated with formaldehyde, tolerance would be decreased and the capacity for unsaturation in the fat stores of ruminants would be increased (Ahmad et al., 2018, p. 2169). Many research studies have focused on various ways of improving the composition of fatty acids in meat because of the integral role that meat plays in human diets, and are aimed at increasing its consumption rate over the years and evaluating the role in human health. The composition of meat fatty acids can be altered by animal diet (feeding), in single-stomach poultry and pigs where the quality of alpha-linolenic, linoleic, and long-chain polyunsaturated fatty acids unexpectedly react to high dietary applications. Important variations were observed between the fatty acid composition of grain and pasture-fed animals, giving a higher polyunsaturated fatty acid concentration in the pasture-fed animal groups (Ahmad et al., 2018, p. 2169). This proves once again how important it is to stick to organic meat and the benefits of refraining from consuming grain-fed animals.

Minerals

Minerals are often identified as the nutrients found in consumable food materials that lack any amount of carbon and are essential for proper physical growth and development as well as preserving the human body. They are split into two nutrient categories i.e., macro- and micro-minerals, on the foundation of their demand by the human body. Macro-minerals are those, which are required by the body in larger amounts (Ahmad et al., 2018, p. 2169). These include minerals like sodium, calcium, phosphorus, magnesium, chloride potassium and sulphur, while micro-minerals refer to minerals that are required in smaller amounts including iron, zinc, iodine, copper, cobalt, manganese, selenium, and fluoride. Potassium is a quantitatively dominant mineral in comparison to others like phosphorus, sodium, and magnesium. Meat is also a primary or dominant source of iron, zinc, and selenium. All of these minerals perform different functions to promote and enable growth, development, and maintenance in the human body (Ahmad et al. 2018, p.2169).

Potassium

Potassium helps the metabolism, nerve impulse transmission, growth, muscle building, and maintaining of acid-base balance in the human body (Ahmad et al., 2018, p. 2169).

Phosphorus

Phosphorus is an important mineral element that provides energy, forms phospholipids along with calcium, which also involves the formation of bones and teeth (Ahmad et al., 2018, p. 2169).

Sodium

Sodium regulates and controls the water content in the body, and it also aids in the transport of CO_2 and maintains the osmotic pressure of body fluids (Ahmad et al., 2018, p. 2169).

Magnesium

Magnesium repairs and improves the growth of the human body, maintains blood pressure, stops tooth decay, and helps to keep the bones dense and healthy (Ahmad et al., 2018, p. 2169).

Zinc

Zinc forms parts of many enzymes required for the body's immune system, and it also plays a role in cell division, growth, and wound healing (Ahmad et al., 2018, p. 2169).

Selenium

Selenium prevents cancer, regulates the poisonous effect of heavy metals, and helps the body digest and recover after vaccinations (Ahmad et al., 2018, p. 2169).

Iron

Iron is one of the key minerals existing in meat and it plays a crucial role in human health and its deficiency causes numerous limitations in the basic functioning of the human body. It particularly disturbs child growth and development. The process of metabolizing iron is quite different from other mineral contents in the sense that it is excreted and more than 90% of it is used internally in the body (Ahmad et al., 2018, p. 2169). A lack of iron and loss of red blood cells gravely impacts the intestines, urinary tract, and skin, and also causes problems during the menstruation period among females especially when they are actively bleeding. An iron deficiency could be treated or prevented by adjusting the diet or supplementing with iron. Iron is accessible through a number of foods and occurs in two forms; heme and nonheme iron. The first one comes from the hemoglobin and myoglobin, meaning that it is found in animal foods primarily and has a high degree of bioavailability that could easily be absorbed in the intestinal lumen (Ahmad et al., 2018, p. 2169).

Meat source	K	Cu	Fe	P	Zn	Mg	Na	Ca
Chopped Mutton, (raw)	244	0.15	0.99	174	4.2	18.8	74	12.5
Chopped Mutton, (grilled)	303	0.25	2.5	205	4.2	22.7	101	17.9

Beef Steak (raw)	335	0.1	2.4	275	4.2	24.4	68	5.5
Beef, Steak (grilled)	369	0.22	3.8	302	5.8	25.1	66	901
Bacon (raw)	267	0.2	1.0	95	2.4	12.2	976	13.6
Bacon, (frie	516	0.2	2.7	228	3.7	25.8	2792	11.6

d)								
Pork (raw)	399	0.1	1.5	224	2.5	26.2	44	4.2
Chopped Pork, (grilled)	259	0.1	2.5	179	3.6	14.8	60	8.2

Organ Meat as a Mineral Source

It has been shown that the offal organs are considerably rich in mineral contents like iron, zinc, and copper, as compared to the minerals that are present in muscular tissues. According to Ahmad et al. (2018, p.2169). Children on a fully vegetarian diet could potentially experience slower cognitive activity due to zinc deficiency, so the importance of meat consumption has been emphasized. Mineral contents of offal organs are depicted in the table below:

Meat source	Fe	P	Na	Ca	Cu	Mg	Zn	K
Ox (Kidney)	5.6	231	182	9	0.5	16	1.8	232
Ox (Liver)	7.1	362	80	6.1	2.4	19.2	4.1	321
Sheep (Liver)	9.5	371	75	7.1	8.8	19.1	4.0	291

| Pig (Kidney) | 5.1 | 272 | 191 | 8.1 | 0.7 | 19.1 | 2.7 | 291 |
| Pig (Liver) | 21.2 | 372 | 88 | 6.2 | 2.8 | 21.3 | 7.0 | 319 |

Vitamins

Vitamins are a group of organic substances that function in a variation of dimensions in the human body. These nutrients are required in moderate or small amounts and are very important for the proper growth, development, and preservation of the human body. They are especially required in the early age of life by children (Ahmad et al., 2018, p. 2169). They partake in various metabolic processes involving a series of chemical and biochemical reactions. One of their distinguishing features is that they generally cannot be prepared by the mammalian cells, so must be supplied through the diet (Ahmad et al., 2018, p. 2169). They are commonly divided into two groups on the basis of their ability to dissolve in water and fat as solvents. These are known as water soluble vitamins and fat-soluble vitamins. Water soluble vitamins include the B-complex vitamins (thiamine, riboflavin, nicotinic acid, pyridoxine, choline, biotin, folic acid, cyanocobalamin, inositol, vitamin B6 and vitamin B12) and vitamin C (Ahmad et al., 2018, p. 2169). Fat soluble vitamins of meat including vitamin A, vitamin D, and vitamin K, also contribute to the nutritional significance of meat. Meat is a good nutritional source that contains 5 of the B-complex vitamins including thiamine, riboflavin, nicotinic acid, vitamin B6, and vitamin B12. It also contains pantothenic acid and biotin, but a weak amount of folacin (Ahmad et al., 2018, p. 2169). The vitamin content of various raw meats is illustrated in the table below:

Vitamin units/100 g raw meat	Beef	Bacon	Mutton	Veal	Pork
A (Inter. Unit.)	Trace	Trace	Trace	Trace	Trace
D (Inter. Unit.)	Trace	Trace	Trace	Trace	Trace
B_1 (mg)	0.06	0.39	0.14	0.11	1.2

B_2 (mg)	0.21	0.16	0.24	0.26	0.21
Nicotinic acid (mg)	5.1	1.6	4.99	7.1	5.2
Pantothenic acid (mg)	0.5	0.4	0.6	0.5	0.5
Biotin (µg)	2	8	4	6	5
Folic acid (µg)	9	Nil	2	6	2
B_6 (mg)	0.2	0.3	0.3	0.4	0.4
B_{12} (µg)	2	Nil	2	Nil	2
C (mg)	Nil	Nil	Nil	Nil	Nil

Water Soluble Vitamins

Thiamine

Thiamine teams up with other B-complex vitamins to carry out numerous chemical functions that are needed for the growth and maintenance of our bodies. They are involved in the metabolic actions needed for building energy to perform various bodily functions. A deficiency of thiamine could cause reduced appetite, fatigue, constipation, irritability, and depression. Meat in general is a good source of thiamine with special reference to fish which provides larger quantities of it as compared to other meat sources (Ahmad et al., 2018, p. 2169).

Riboflavin

Riboflavin is considered another essential vitamin that aids in the release of energy produced by the major essentials like proteins, fats, and carbohydrates. It also helps us with our eyesight and is good for the skin. It can also act as an aid in absorbing and general consumption of iron and it is essential for transitioning tryptophan to niacin. Poultry meat, lamb and beef are considered among the best sources of riboflavin (Ahmad et al., 2018, p. 2169).

Niacin

Together with other B-vitamins, niacin works interchangeably with intracellular enzyme systems, including those that contribute to energy production. It is most commonly sourced from meat, fish, and poultry. Its deficiency causes the disease known as pellagra, which is characterized by rough or tender skin. Other problems include memory loss, vomiting and diarrhea (Ahmad et al., 2018, p. 2169).

Vitamin B6

Vitamin B6 plays a rather important role in the proper functioning of approximately 100 enzymes that operate or influence the essential chemical reactions in the human body. It contributes to the synthesis of the neurotransmitters and in the synthesis of heme-iron as a component of hemoglobin. Furthermore, it also helps in the synthesis of niacin from tryptophan. Important meaty sources of vitamin B6 are fish, poultry and meat (Ahmad et al., 2018, p. 2169).

Vitamin B12

This vitamin is important for the synthesis of deoxyribonucleic acid (DNA), which is a gene-containing component of the cell's nucleus, vital for proper growth and development of the human body (Ahmad et al., 2018, p. 2169). Vitamin B12 is found mostly in foods of animal origin like meat, eggs, dairy, etc. Therefore, vegans or vegetarians who consume no animal products may be required to supplement their diet with this vitamin. Individuals who have pernicious anemia which is the inability to absorb vitamin B12 from food, who fail to consume vitamin B12, can be treated successfully with injections or similar supplements of vitamin B12. Meats like liver, beef, lamb, and pork are rich sources of this vitamin despite the cut or location in the animal's body. Some other sources are oysters, fish, egg yolk and cheese (Ahmad et al., 2018, p. 2169).

Fat soluble vitamins

Vitamin A is a fat-soluble vitamin essential for the preservation of healthy tissues and for maintaining good vision and eyesight. Green and yellow vegetables provide vitamin A and it occurs in the form of carotene which the body converts into vitamin A (Ahmad et al., 2018, p. 2169). Milk and margarine are often enriched with vitamin A and liver is recommended as the greatest single animal source of vitamin A. It is also a good source of the other fat-digesting vitamins such as vitamin D and vitamin K. Vitamin contents (water and fat soluble) of various offal organs are depicted in the table below (Ahmad et al., 2018, p. 2169):

Meat source	B_1 (mg)	B_2 (mg)	B_3 (mg)	B_6 (µg)	B_9 (µg)	B_{12} (µg)	Vit. C (mg)	Vit. D (µg)	Vit. A (I.U.)
Brain	0.06	0.02	2.99	0.10	6.0	8.9	23.0	Trace	Trace

Sheep's kidney	0.5	1.9	8.4	0.32	31.0	54.9	6.9	Nil	99
Ox's kidney	0.38	2.2	6.1	0.33	77.2	31.2	10.1	Nil	150
Pig's kidney	0.33	2.0	7.4	0.24	42.1	14.2	14.3	Nil	110
Shee	0.28	3.4	14.1	0.43	220	83	9.9	0.49	20,00

p's liver								0
Ox's liver	0.22	3.2	13.5	0.84	330	109.7	23.0	1.14	17,000
Pig's liver	0.32	3.1	14.7	0.69	110	24.8	13.2	1.14	10,000
Sheep's lung	0.13	0.5	4.8	Nil	Nil	4.8	31.2	Nil	Nil

| Ox's lung | 0.10 | 0.4 | 4.1 | Nil | Nil | 3.2 | 38.7 | Nil | Nil |
| Pig's lung | 0.10 | 0.3 | 3.3 | Nil | Nil | Nil | 13.1 | Nil | Nil |

This concludes that meat and meat products play a significant role in the fulfilment and maintenance of human health. Studies indicated that strong nutritional composition (fats, proteins, and carbohydrates) with minerals, vitamins, and other functional composites play a preventive role against major and minor nutrient deficiency-based illnesses and issues (Ahmad et al., 2018, p. 2169). Meat as a food substance must be included as a significant portion in your diet to meet the required health benefits. Proteins and amino acids are beneficial for growth and the building of muscles in humans. Additionally, minerals and vitamins, including zinc, iron, selenium, sodium, copper, magnesium, calcium, potassium, phosphorus, and vitamin A, along with ample amount of B complex vitamins, are considered as central constituents of meat and are beneficial for overall human health levels (Ahmad et al.,

2018, p. 2169). Now that you know the significant role that meat plays in your overall health as a human, you can approach your carnivore journey with hope and ease.

Conclusion

Hopefully by now, this book has provided you with a better understanding of the carnivore diet as a whole and how it can benefit your life and your mental well-being. As you work through the guidelines and all of the information found throughout the chapters, you should be able to gain a certain perspective that will provide the tools you will need to execute all of the levels of the carnivore diet. Changing your bad habits and going full carnivore is often a very intense practice, especially when you have to cut carbohydrates out of your life completely. It is normal to feel overwhelmed at first, but in due time, you will get the hang of it and become more confident as days go by. Changing your ways is not always as easy; however, you will now be able to improve your health with the help of the carnivore lifestyle and the knowledge that Fox Wild has shared with you.

These resources provided to you in this book can free you from the burden of dealing with dietary issues, health issues, and some of the problems that you may be experiencing mentally. If you have tried fad diets in the past or some of those 30-day challenges, then you already know that they do not work as successfully or sustainably as you would have hoped. Now you know that it was not necessarily your fault, but it was mainly because of the restriction of your caloric intake, which left you deprived of the nutrients that your body and mind needed to function properly. You might have been a bit clueless about the low-carb/high-fat approach and just needed a little push in the right direction. Well, here you are now, fully capable and ready to take on the challenge that will eventually become a big part of your everyday life.

Yes, you may have been a victim of the false hope that invasive or strict diets sometimes proclaim. Now is your chance to start saying "hell no" to fads, starvation, deprivation, and countless disappointing results. You have now been formally introduced to the concept of the carnivore diet and you have the basic principles at hand. With all of this information, you are also more informed about the importance of following in the footsteps of our early ancestors and realize how important protein is for your body, mind, and arguably, your spirit too. Meat eating was essential for evolution since the day that humans came into existence, so this diet is nothing but natural and instinctive, to say the least.

Surely, the idea of cutting carbohydrates out of your life forever is no picnic. It can be a very intimidating and invasive thought; however, you should think of it as a way to nourish and feed your body, instead of feeling like something is being taken away from you. You are not losing out; you are gaining so much more than you can comprehend. You are worthy of a good life and the carnivore lifestyle can help you to achieve it. Although you have been told your entire life that a healthy diet consists of plant-based carbohydrates, what have these plants and plant products actually done for you? They are not essential for survival. They might not be bad for you in any way, but they are definitely not keeping you alive or doing you any favors at this point.

Take your time when you are working through the three levels of the carnivore diet and give yourself enough time to adjust to each one accordingly. You will be changing many aspects of your life for the better, so it is not going to happen overnight. Be patient, committed, and fierce. It is time for you to take back your life and nourish your body and mind. Much of what is discussed throughout this book is based on the testimonials of real people who struggled with real problems until they found the healing hand of the carnivore diet. Leave sugar, in all its forms, completely alone. Fat is not your enemy, but sugar is. You will soon come to realize how much mental clarity and wellness you can experience and the thought of reintroducing sugar into your life will cease to exist.

Follow the recipes in this book and be as adventurous and experimental as you can before reaching Level 3. You will notice how eating all of these protein-rich meals will dampen your urge to binge on sugary snacks or treats. It will nourish your body and mind as well as keep you full and energized. Surely, everyone feels a bit down and out during the transition phase, but once you are over that hurdle, you will start to feel the benefits almost immediately. There is a reason why so many people trust in this process and why it has gained so much popularity over the years. It works, it is safe, sustainable, realistic, and healthy. Plan your meals ahead of time and create weekly menus and shopping lists. You do not have to cook each meal separately; it can be a seemingly effortless experience if you learn how to utilize meal preparation and planning.

Start small and work your way up gradually. Going in headfirst at lightning speed will only cause a big crash and you will be less likely to succeed and reach your goals. Instead, work at a gradual pace and trust whatever your body is trying to tell you. Try not to eat lean meats or any fruits and vegetables once you are fully submerged in the lifestyle, as doing so could mess with ketosis and fat-burning stages. Be patient and trust the process.

It is far more respected to reach your goals than you may have first imagined. In addition to the fact that you will live a healthier life, you will decrease your chances of experiencing frightening and potentially fatal illnesses and ailments. There is no challenging the fact that your physical appearance will also be a factor; however, carrying on with a lengthy and optimistic life should consistently and ultimately be your main goal and objective. The well-being of your body and mind are connected to one another, and it is substantial for carnivores to understand that your gut health can impact your mental health. When you understand how beneficial the carnivore lifestyle can be for your well-being, it ought to serve as a spark or driver behind your will to change and get rid of bad habits.

You are now capable of changing your life by means of what you put in your body. You are in charge and it is possible for you to grab this opportunity and bring it on home. You are worthy, capable, and soon you will be a strong and healthy individual too. For more success stories to inspire and motivate you on your journey, follow this link: https://meatrx.com/category/success-stories/. If you found this book helpful, insightful, and likeable, please leave a review on Amazon and tell us more about your experience. You can also join the online forum here: https://www.reddit.com/r/zerocarb/.

References

Ahmad, R. S., Imran, A., and Hussain, M. B. (2018). Nutritional composition of meat. *Meat science and nutrition*, 2169–2170. https://doi.org/10.5772/intechopen.77045

Connor, T. (2014, December 11). *Circadian rhythms: You are when you eat*. The Paleo Diet®. https://thepaleodiet.com/eat-circadian-rhythms

Corporate Wellness Magazine. (n.d.). *6 Tips to differentiate hunger vs. thirst*. Retrieved December 20, 2020, from https://www.corporatewellnessmagazine.com/article/hunger-vs-thirst

Diet, T. L. P. (2020, July 29). *Circadian rhythms: You are when you eat*. The Paleo Diet®. https://thepaleodiet.com/eat-circadian-rhythms

Fetters, A. K., and Grieger, L. R. (2020, October 19). *Incomplete vs. complete protein: What's the difference? | Everyday Health*. EverydayHealth.Com. https://www.everydayhealth.com/diet-nutrition/incomplete-vs-complete-protein-whats-the-difference/

Gunnars, K. B. (2019, March 8). *10 Science-backed reasons to eat more protein*. Healthline. https://www.healthline.com/nutrition/10-

reasons-to-eat-more-
protein#TOC_TITLE_HDR_2

Hyson, S. (2020, May 15). *The carnivore diet: Is eating only meat healthy, or totally f@#$ing crazy?* Onnit Academy. https://www.onnit.com/academy/the-carnivore-diet/

Is it possible? (n.d.). CarniWay.Nyc. Retrieved December 2, 2020, from https://www.carniway.nyc/is-it-possible

Joseph, M. (2019, November 13). *Can too much protein cause kidney damage?* Nutrition Advance. https://www.nutritionadvance.com/too-much-protein-kidney-damage/

Lazzaris, S. (2020, October 30). *Does sugar damage our health?* Food Unfolded. https://www.foodunfolded.com/article/does-sugar-damage-our-health?gclid=Cj0KCQiAifz-BRDjARIsAEElyGJUJw8__GSOxF55jCWT19 6Ny4s-YcuDS6QLKOTLHdjANS4C6Tz9OcEaAgJ8E ALw_wcB

La Fleur, E. (2015, April 20). V*itamin C. Eat meat. Drink water.* https://zerocarbzen.com/vitamin C/plants - zerocarb. (2010, September 30).

Mayo Clinic. (2019, August 15). *Chronic kidney disease - Symptoms and causes.*

https://www.mayoclinic.org/diseases-conditions/chronic-kidney-disease/symptoms-causes/syc-20354521

McBroom, P. (1999, June 14). 06.14.99 - *Meat-eating was essential for human evolution, says UC Berkeley anthropologist specializing in diet.* University of California, Berkeley. https://www.berkeley.edu/news/media/releases/99legacy/6-14-1999a.html

MeatRx,.(2029, December 16). Success stories. https://meatrx.com/category/success-stories/

Midhani, R. (2018, October 5). *Beef cuts explained: Your ultimate guide to different cuts of beef.* Fine Dining Lovers. https://www.finedininglovers.com/article/beef-cuts-explained

Miller, A. M. (2019, January 29). *What to know about the carnivore diet.* U.S. News. https://health.usnews.com/wellness/food/articles/2019-01-29/what-is-the-carnivore-diet

Norton, R. S. D. (2020, October 1). *Keto vs. carnivore diet: Which one is better? –.* KissMyKetoBlog. https://blog.kissmyketo.com/articles/keto-diet-basics/keto-vs-carnivore-which-one-is-better/

Phelps, N. (2020, November 7). *Carnivore diet: A beginner's guide to an all-meat diet.* Chomps, https://chomps.com/blogs/news/carnivore-diet

Ratini, M. (2020, April 7). *The truth about sugar addiction.* WebMD. https://www.webmd.com/diet/ss/slideshow-sugar-addiction

Reddit.
https://www.reddit.com/r/zerocarb/wiki/plants

Roberts Stoler, D. (2015, June 9). *The power of protein to optimize brain health.* PSYCHOLOGY TODAY. https://www.onnit.com/academy/the-carnivore-diet/

Sisson, M. (2020, October 27). *Carnivore diet: What the research says* | Mark's Daily Apple.Mark'sDailyApple. https://www.marksdailyapple.com/carnivore-diet-research-science/#ref-27

Statham, T. (n.d.). CarniWay. CarniWay.Nyc. Retrieved December 6, 2020, from https://www.carniway.nyc/*carnivorous-way-of-eating*

Stock, K. (2018). *The ultimate 30-day guide to going full carnivore.* Meat Health. https://meat.health/wp-content/uploads/2018/02/The-Ultimate-30-Day-Guide-to-Going-Full-Carnivore.pdf

Streit, M. L. S. (2019, August 26). *All you need to know about the carnivore (all-meat) diet*. Healthline. https://www.healthline.com/nutrition/carnivore-diet

Truong, K. (2020, December 11). *Why is sleep so important to weight loss?* Sleep Foundation. https://www.sleepfoundation.org/physical-health/weight-loss-and-sleep

Watson, M. (2020, September 17). *From belly to trotter— All the pork cuts you could hope to cook*. The Spruce Eats. https://www.thespruceeats.com/complete-guide-to-pork-cuts-4067791

Why is Protein important in your diet? | Piedmont Healthcare. (n.d.). Piedmont Healthcare. Retrieved November 30, 2020, from https://www.piedmont.org/living-better/why-is-protein-important-in-your-diet

Woods, T. (2020a, September 17). *How to start the carnivore diet – 20 Experts share their tips*. Carnivore Style. https://carnivorestyle.com/20-experts-share-their-tips-on-the-carnivore-diet/

Woods, T. (2020b, October 30). *What is the carnivore diet? How to get started on lifestyle*. Carnivore Style. https://carnivorestyle.com/carnivore-diet/

Woods, T. (2020, October 4). *What's the best carnivore diet supplement?* Review and Buyers Guide. Carnivore

Style. https://carnivorestyle.com/carnivore-diet/supplements/

Lightning Source UK Ltd.
Milton Keynes UK
UKHW051526290821
389628UK00012B/275